THE DIET WARS!

Decisions That Have Harmed the Health of Millions

by

John M. Raht

ISBN-13: 978-1469954752 (CreateSpace-Assigned)

ISBN-10: 1469954753

John M. Raht, P.O. Box 9, Naalehu, HI 96772

Phone: 808-929-8723   Email: johnraht@aol.com

To Julie for her years of love and friendship,

To Barbara, a caring mother,

To Dave, for his strength and support,

To Ann, who made it happen,

And finally to the fond memory of Chuck.

Contents

WHAT HAPPENED?

Something has gone very wrong. In the last 50 years millions have had their health seriously damaged by following diet plans recommended by authorities. And it didn't need to happen. No, it was not some terrorist plot or a deliberate act to cause health problems. It was caused by mistakes made by the very people and institutions that we trust. And the sad part is that they thought they were doing the right thing.

But look at what has happened. As an example, look at the weight increase in the general population from 1981 to 1991. In 1981, 8.6% of the population was overweight and 4.1% was obese. Ten years later this had increased to 22.4% overweight and 13.7% obese. That is an overall increase of almost 300%! This increase was even greater in the 30- to 50-year-olds. And that weight increase continued. Why? These people didn't suddenly make a major decrease in their physical activity or any other behavior that could account for this but one. A major change in diet.

This book is not a tabloid exposé of major conspiracies or a startling uncovering of evildoers. It is instead an attempt to explain how things got the way they are in the field of nutrition and how destructive this has been for a large number of people. Just look around you. While following the guidelines of both the United States Government and most of the departments of nutrition in colleges and universities,

1

problems like obesity, diabetes, and other diet-related diseases have increased dramatically. Dr. Robert H. Lustig from the University of California has pointed out that the latest generation will probably have a shorter life span than their parents for the first time in our nation's history. By 2030, at the present rate of increase, one-third of the population will have diabetes as well as other weight-related health issues. Studies reflect this increase. From 1980 to 2008, the obesity rate in children six to eleven years of age increased from 6.5% to 19.6% and is still increasing.

This book is an attempt to show you how and why things went wrong. To do this we will examine diet books, diet research, and diet programs that have been prominent during the last half-century and look at the promises, practices, and pitfalls they contain.

If, over the last few years, you have tried to follow a healthy eating plan, you know that there is more than a little confusion and conflict as to what is best. The following are some of the statements commonly found in professional directives and popular diet books:

A. Calories in, calories out. Years ago, a biologist at UCLA told me that this would make perfect sense if you had a test tube in your belly and a Bunsen burner up your butt. But you don't, and as a specific guide to eating, it has a number of problems.

B. Simply overeating is the cause of all overweight problems. That sounds obvious but may not be even close to the whole story.

C. Fat people simply eat more than thin people. They usually don't. In fact most of them eat the same amount or even less than people of normal weight.

D. The nutrition departments in our universities have always been the best source for healthy eating guidelines. Sadly, this often has not been true.

E. The United States Government's new "Eating Plan" is a specific guide that should show you how to eat wisely. Many people disagree. Some well respected experts regard it as something of a political joke.

F. And finally, have you noticed that the most successful diet books of the last thirty years have not been written by nutritional experts, but by people in completely different fields? For example Deirdre Barrett, Ph.D., who wrote *Waistland*, is a psychologist at Harvard Medical School. Barry Sears, Ph.D., who wrote *The Zone*, is a research scientist. Dean Ornish, M.D., who wrote *The Spectrum*, is a heart specialist. Robert Atkins, author of *Dr. Atkins' Diet Revolution* and other books, was a cardiologist, as is Dr. Arthur Agatston, who wrote *The South Beach Diet*. Actress Suzanne Somers wrote *Eat Great, Lose Weight*. A currently popular diet book is *You: On A Diet* written by Mehmet Oz, who was trained as a heart surgeon, and Michael Roizen, an anesthesiologist. And the list goes on.

Why I Wrote This Book

My credentials for this project are very different from those of most others in the field of nutrition. Briefly, my background goes from college textbook acquisitions editor for a major publisher, to the West Coast Manager of the Education Department of the National Broadcasting Company. Following that, I started my own organization evaluating and marketing documentaries and other materials for universities, libraries, and schools. A large part of all of these jobs was evaluation. As acquisitions editor, I developed a number of college textbooks in the areas of English, mathematics, physical anthropology and most importantly, regarding this book, cultural anthropology. Later at NBC, my job involved the evaluation and marketing of documentaries for use everywhere from elementary to graduate school.

So how did all of this prepare me for writing a book about nutrition? My interest in the field of diet and nutrition started years ago while working with cultural anthropologists. Food, how it is grown, killed, or gathered, has a strong cultural impact. I grew up over eighty years ago in the back country of Arizona, where hunting for meat and some wild food plants was still a standard thing to do. I was surprised at how often those same food practices could be found in other cultures. What people ate and how it impacted their health became both a professional and personal interest.

But there was also a far more personal reason. In 1962, at the age of 34, I had what the doctor called a "stress-related event." Not a heart attack but enough of a scare to get my full attention. I was lucky in that my doctor (sadly, I can't recall his name) was ahead of his time regarding the subject of an overall plan for good health. At the time my personal habits were not that sterling. I had come of age in the late 1940s when smoking two packs a day and lifting few things heavier than a stiff drink was about the standard behavior for many men, myself included.

The doctor questioned me in depth about my habits and family history. He pointed out that my health history was not encouraging. Most men in my family had died in their fifties or early sixties of cancer or heart disease. The women lived longer but also had heart trouble. The doctor pointed out that putting that family history together with my smoking, poor diet, and lack of exercise meant that the odds were very good that I wouldn't make it to 60. So I quit smoking (not easy!) and started to pay much more attention to diet and exercise. He said that by doing all of this I might make it until I was 70. As I write this I am 83 and still going.

The end result of the health problem that happened in 1962 was this: Whereas before I had only an academic interest in good health, it now became a much more personal one. And by luck I was in an ideal position to pursue that interest.

Back when I started in college textbook publishing, it was a far different industry than it is today. In the late 1950s and early 1960s, when I visited a university campus, I was seen as someone who could discuss new ideas and share the latest gossip, as well as liberally provide free books. This meant that my interest in dietary practices could be discussed not only with people in the departments of nutrition but also professors in subjects like chemistry, biology, and as mentioned before, anthropology.

During that time I watched the changes, some sensible and some almost bizarre, that were happening in the field of diet. This led me to the habit of evaluating the different books on nutrition and diet as one eating plan or another became popular. Because of over 50 years of watching the "diet wars" and talking to some of the top people in the areas of the scientific disciplines that impact nutrition, over time I became more and more concerned about the conflicts and misinformation in this debate. And so this book.

What I will try to do is show you how this controversy developed over the years, the problems it caused, and how you can use this information to help you make better decisions regarding your own health. I think the best way to do this is to start with brief reviews of many of the books on diet and health that have come along during the last half-century. Very quickly it becomes apparent that the experts in the field of diet don't agree. Or in many cases don't just disagree but do so to the point of name calling and heated arguments.

I will try to give a thumbnail sketch of several books that look at various sides of this debate. Using these books and others as a starting point, we will try to get some answers. And these answers are desperately needed if we are to address the health problems, stemming from poor eating and exercise habits, that are all too common today. As we look at these books, I will often suggest that you borrow a book and read a part that I feel is of particular importance. There are cases where you might even think it wise to buy the book. Since it's your health that is the real subject here, building a collection of books for reference can be of real help.

So let's take look at those books.

BOOK REVIEWS

DR. ATKINS' DIET REVOLUTION

Dr. Robert C. Atkins.

Probably the best place to start is with the famous (or infamous, depending on your point of view) book that made the low-carbohydrate diet a big hit with the general public. This book, first published in 1972 and updated ten years later as *Dr. Atkins' New Diet Revolution*, was the first well-known book on what would become a popular type of diet plan. The standard take on this type of diet is that it is a "new craze." It wasn't. In fact, it could probably be traced back to a type of eating used by the athletes of ancient Greece when they were preparing for their games.

One of the first publications in more modern times to take this approach can be found in *Letters On Corpulence*, by William Bunting, published in 1864. It, like Atkins, also got all kinds of flack from the medical community of the time, not unlike the vehement objections regarding this type of eating plan that can still be heard today. In fact, the objections to this approach has gotten to the point that some of the newer low-carb diet books spend a lot of time explaining why they are not "really" low-carb. Another popular book in this group is *The South Beach Diet*. It starts out in its very first sentence stating "The South Beach Diet is not low-carb." This is more than a bit of a stretch, but more on that later.

Back to Atkins' first book. Because people found his system did work, this book ended up selling millions of copies, causing it to quickly become the most successful diet book as well as the diet book most reviled by many "experts" in the diet field. Read page one, and you can see why. Atkins writes that most people think that overweight is caused by overeating. But he continues, "Not so! This is one of those assumptions we have always taken for granted, one of the many myths about overweight that it is now time to unlearn." He states that most overweight is caused by a metabolic imbalance that his diet can correct. He also writes that his is a no-hunger diet. He says that people eat 2000-3000 calories a day on his plan and still lose weight. But most people, he says, will eat less because the food eaten does a better job of satisfying hunger. He writes that the calorie-counting approach has failed and then takes a hard swipe at his own profession by pointing out that despite this failure the medical profession has not searched widely for alternatives. Instead, there has been a flood of low-calorie food and drink products, and the drug industry has produced a "Niagara" (his word) of diet pills, all of which have failed to do the job.

Next he writes that a problem too often overlooked is the diseases caused by what he calls a carbohydrate intolerance. He claims that such problems as overweight, diabetes, hypoglycemia, and others can be traced to this condition. He feels that one of the reasons more attention hasn't been paid to problems with refined carbohydrates is the large sums of money being poured into the various departments of nutrition by the manufacturers of refined carbohydrate foodstuffs. He also believes that another cause of this weight problem is a sugar addiction. He points out that we now consume more sugar in two weeks than we did in a year just two centuries ago.

Atkins says that we evolved mainly on a diet of meat and that's what our bodies were built to handle. Back then we only ate small amounts of carbohydrates and all of those were unrefined. Only in the last few centuries have we switched to highly-refined carbohydrates. At the top of page six he makes an interesting statement regarding carbohydrates, "One of the reasons that it (his diet) is remarkably effective is that when you take away carbs you take away hunger." Another impressive quote comes from a textbook on the diseases of metabolism edited by Dr. Philip K. Bondy, who was Chairman of the Department of Internal Medicine at Yale Medical School at the time. Dr. Bondy says that no carbohydrate is required in the diet. He goes on to state "it has been shown experimentally that human beings can survive in good health for months on a diet of meat and fat."

At the beginning of Chapter Two Atkins gets down to the nitty-gritty of his plan. You don't count calories or eat almost any carbs to start. He tells how other low-carb diets (he names several) are all a step in the right direction but there is a vital difference with his plan. Most of the other diet plans tell you to cut carbs down to 60 grams a day. This way the body will not throw off ketones. Ketones in the urine or breath is considered a problem by many physicians, a viewpoint which Atkins says is dead wrong. He feels that this problem comes, in part, from the confusion between ketosis and ketoacidosis, which is an indication of a problem.

And right here is where we get to the part that made this plan so popular: You get to pee on a stick! You buy these things called Ketostix, and by checking your urine with this stick, you find out if you are producing ketones as wanted. I'm serious when I say that this urination test for the ketones factor gives his diet a big leg up over other plans. On other diets you wait to see the scales register less or the tape measure show that your belly has shrunk. But with the "pee on a stick" approach not only can you tell very quickly if you're winning, but it's also a great way to monitor your progress. He says that when the stick is purple that also means that you are producing FMH (which stands for Fat Mobilization Hormones), which is what you want. He gives a long description of what this is and why it works. He says that to produce FMH is the whole purpose of this diet. There is a bit of a problem with FMH . I haven't run across this anywhere else. Also in the revised edition of this book, it doesn't show up at all. This seems a bit strange because he makes a big deal out of why it is what you are after. He says it is a product of the pituitary gland and was first discovered by three researchers in England in 1960. More about this when I get to his revision of this book where FMH disappears and is replaced with FMS which stands for "fat-mobilizing substance."

Anyhow, you stay with eating almost no carbs until the stick turns purple. Then you add carbs until you lose the color and back up until you get it back. This gives you a day-to-day check on your progress. In his book he gives a great deal of background information before getting to the diet itself in Chapter Twelve.

Like many of today's diet gurus, Dr. Atkins is not a fan of processed foods. Unlike some of the others, however, he gives the background of how they developed and the logical reasons they were necessary in the first place. It's a simple matter of storage. If you polish rice or de-germinate and bleach flour you greatly increase its shelf life. When humans changed from hunter-gatherers to farmers this ability to store food was a major advantage. Then it's on to considering sugar. It's no surprise that like most others, Atkins feels that sugar in almost any form is not part of a healthy diet.

The big disagreement he had with most people in the diet field when he first wrote this book was his argument that calories are not the key to weight gain or loss. One of several examples he gives for his belief is a study done in the Berkeley, California School System in 1968. I thought this was interesting. Ruth L. Hueneman followed the daily calorie intake of 950 students from the ninth to twelfth grade. She took both dietary histories and body measurements. The average calories eaten by boys that were of average weight was over 3,000. For average-weight girls it was 2,060 calories. The average intake of overweight boys was only 2,360 calories and overweight girls averaged only 1,530. The study goes on to point out that in the three years that were covered, there were no glaring exceptions. During this time both the overweight girls and overweight boys got fatter! Many of the other studies Atkins quotes come up with this same conclusion: So, he says, it's not just about the calories.

The rest of the book outlines his diet in detail as well as listing day-to-day eating plans, recipes and some questions and answers, which is much the same thing that you find in most diet books. One thing that seems strange today is that he makes little comment on the effects, good or bad, regarding saturated fats. The easy answer to this might be that when he was writing this book, saturated fats were no big deal. But that's not completely true, so I don't know why he didn't give it more coverage.

Two final comments about this book. The first: on page 143, he casually states, "You may notice a change (a slight diminution) in the bowel pattern because of the lack of roughage." I found this to be a monstrous understatement! After ten days on the diet, I found that elimination started to approach the equivalent of childbirth. Constipation is much too mild a term to describe the experience. So I believe that some type of fiber supplement is a wise addition if you try this diet. Another thing worth mentioning is a comment he makes about eating fruit. On page 148 he says "nothing in the diet up to this point is as likely to stop your progress dead as is fruit." This sounds strange, but I kept running across this same idea in several other diet books. If they didn't warn about fruit, when they made their meal suggestions fruit was strangely absent.

OK, now a quick look at the revision.

DR. ATKINS' NEW DIET REVOLUTION

Dr. Robert C. Atkins

Dr. Atkins wrote several other books such as *Dr Atkins' Quick and Easy New Diet Cookbook* and *Dr. Atkins' Age-defying Diet Revolution*, but the real second edition of his first book is *Dr. Atkins' NEW Diet Revolution*. So that is the next diet book we'll examine.

This new book has pretty much the same approach as the first one. However, the criticism that he received over the years may be the reason for some of the changes. For example, he apologizes for being too harsh on the low-fat crowd, saying that "they were sincere in their efforts to help people." Another change from the first book is that this time he doesn't get all worked up over what he called the "calorie hoax" as he did in the first edition. In fact, he says on page 17 that "it is true that gaining weight results from taking in more calories than you expend." But you can't stop there because he adds what he calls a gigantic "but." And it is: "But this only happens when you mix carbs with fat."

In this edition he puts an even bigger emphasis on what he calls "metabolic disturbance" involving insulin problems. Part of the problem, he says, comes from things like the Food Guide Pyramid created by the U.S. Department of Agriculture. Here he is referring to the old food guide, not the new one, although I doubt he would have been wild about the new one either. If you have examined the new Federal Diet Plan, you might agree it still has some major problems, but more on that later. Anyhow, putting together the metabolic disturbance factor and the insulin problem, he adds them up to what he calls the primary problem with most overweight people and that is that they are carbohydrate-sensitive.

Once again, Atkins feels that the basic villains are refined carbohydrates and the worst of these are sugar, high-fructose corn syrup, white flour, and the products they contain. He points out that between 1910 and 1970 there was an escalation in heart problems in our country that nicely parallels the increase in consumption of refined carbohydrates. He makes the comparison, which you hear quite often, to the French diet. French men of the 1960s ate about the same amount of meat and fish that we did, four times the butter, and twice as much cheese, but had much lower rates of stroke and heart disease. French women did even better, having the lowest heart disease rate in the Western world. The key he says? Lower refined carbs.

In Chapter Five he goes into the insulin problem at some length. The big factor here is controlling blood-sugar levels. He states flatly that you can't control insulin properly without eating fat.

In Chapter Six we get back to ketosis, only now he calls it "lipolysis." He says he is using this term now because too many people confused ketosis with diabetic ketoacidosis, which is a product of disease. It is lipolysis that makes it possible to lose weight without the hunger found in low-calorie diets. In this edition he gives more background information on the research that has been done on this subject.

Another new factor in this edition is his coverage of the "net carb" idea. This has cropped up in the last few years with the popularity of different low-carb diets. Basically it is taking into account the effect of fiber on blood sugar. He uses the example of a cookie made with white flour and a couple of fiber-rich crackers, both equaling ten grams of carbs. The big difference is that the cookie puts all ten grams into the blood stream, but since the crackers have four grams of fiber included in their ten grams of carbs you only get six grams of carbs that get to the system as the fiber isn't digestible.

Also new in this edition is a discussion of the Glycemic Index. This is an index that tells you how fast glucose from a given food enters the bloodstream after it is eaten. He points out that this index has not been standardized as yet but is still a good guide as to how different foods affect blood sugar. Atkins isn't the only diet writer who uses this index. If it becomes more standardized, I think that you will start to see it used like carb and calorie lists are today. Atkins says that the Harvard Nurses' Study (a well-known study tracking the dietary and health habits of 75,521 nurses for many years) shows that consumption of carbs with a high Glycemic Index was strongly associated with an increase in heart disease.

On page 90 Atkins makes a point that I think should have been given more stress. He says that he does not agree with lumping together fruits and vegetables as being essentially equal in benefits. He points out that vegetables have more antioxidant per carbohydrate gram than fruits and so are more valuable in the diet.

In Chapter Nine, "Facts and Fallacies About the Atkins Nutritional Approach," he finally takes on the saturated-fat debate. (But for some reason the term "saturated fat"can't be found in the index.) He says that the Framingham study, another one of the big health studies, showed that people with the highest intake of saturated fat had 76% fewer strokes than those with the lowest intake.

In Chapter Eleven he gives the twelve rules that he says you must follow to make the diet work. This is a more specific prescription than is found in the first edition and probably easier to follow. Finally, what I think is the big plus for this edition over the first one is the way he treats exercise. He gives it its own chapter. It's Chapter Twenty-two, "Exercise: Its Non-Negotiable." Over the fourteen pages of this chapter he outlines different approaches and programs. But in all of them his message is clear — "Get moving!"

Something that should be added here is the book *The All-new Atkins Advantage* by Stuart L. Trager, M.D. with Colette Heimowitz, M.Sc., published in 2007. Despite the name there are several suggestion that don't parallel Atkins. A push for fiber, an emphasis on omega-3s, and more attention to what they call "a proportional, reasonable intake of other healthy fats" is a bit different that the original Atkins approach.

The basis of this book is a twelve-week program of diet and exercise which seems to be well thought out. Also a nice point is their stress on eating organic products as well as meat and dairy products that are raised in a natural way without a lot of hormones, antibiotics, nitrates, and other preservatives.

Sadly, the "pee on a stick" plan of the original Atkins is missing.

THE SOUTH BEACH DIET

Arthur Agatston, M.D.

The next logical entry of the better known low-carbohydrate diet books would be this one. The subtitle of this book says that it's *The Delicious, Doctor-Designed, Foolproof Plan for Fast and Healthy Weight Loss*. Wow! As I mentioned before, the book's first sentence reads, "The South Beach Diet is not low-carb." This is a pretty big stretch. The next sentence states, "Nor is it low-fat." At this point you might feel that he has pretty much boxed himself in until he adds that instead it is all about the "right" carbs and the "right" fats.

Still, on page one he says that you'll eat normal-sized helpings of meat, chicken, turkey, fish, and shellfish as well as eggs, cheese, nuts and salads with real olive oil in the dressing. And it gets better. He says that on his plan you'll eat three balanced meals a day and you'll eat until your hunger is satisfied. You will also have snacks mid-morning and mid-afternoon whether you need them or not. And to top it off, you'll have dessert after dinner!

But wait, come over to the dark side, which shows up on page 4. For the first two weeks of this diet you won't consume bread, rice, potatoes, pasta, baked goods, fruit, candy, cake, cookies, ice cream, alcohol, or any kind of sugar. After two weeks, things start to ease up a bit. But look closely at those first two weeks: It's pretty much an Atkins diet look-alike with one big, a very big, exception. And that exception is the restriction of saturated fat. This is the reason, I think, that this book was accepted by the medical community far better than many of the other low-carb diets that don't restrict this type of fat. But since the thrust of this plan is the restriction of saturated fats why isn't there more discussion as to why?

But let's move on to another interesting statement. It's the first sentence of Chapter Two. Here he writes, "I'm not a diet doctor." This has to give one pause, but he then explains that he's a heart doctor who got disillusioned with the standard low-fat diets that were being touted by most of the experts. The reason for his disillusionment was that these diets simply did not work over the long term. And that is when he started studying diets. He found that the medical literature was starting to discuss more and more something called the "insulin resistance syndrome" and its effect on obesity and heart health. He explains that this insulin resistance is why the body stores too much fat, especially in the mid-section. He points out, as do many others in this field, that we are animals designed to store fat as protection against famine. The problem is that we did away with the famine side of the equation. About here he makes the statement that more and more people are starting to agree with. He writes: "Much of our excess weight comes from the carbohydrates we eat, especially the highly processed ones found in baked goods like cakes, breads, snacks, and other convenient favorites." He says that decreasing the intake of these foods can clear up insulin resistance.

And it is here where he tells us why his diet is so superior to the Atkins plan. As you might have guessed, it's the matter of saturated fat. He claims that Atkins bans virtually all carbohydrates and leaves the dieter to exist mostly on proteins. He goes on to point out that Atkins permits limitless saturated fats. These are, "as most people know" (his statement), the bad fats. And he goes on to say that if you eat the Atkins way, your blood chemistry "might suffer." The use of the word "might" is wise on his part because most of the more recent research shows just the opposite. He adds, "Not everyone wants to give up vegetables, fruit, bread and pasta forever." It's hard to know the source of this statement as I haven't found this prescription in either Atkins or any other diet book. He says that he recognizes that there will be days when "you just need that chocolate ice cream or lemon meringue pie." You have to wonder if he feels that there are also days when you just have to have diabetes or heart disease. Probably not. I think the best thing to do is stop and take a good hard look at your "needs." After discussing Atkins, he then moves on to claim that Dr. Berry Sears' book, *The Zone*, is too complex and burdensome.

In the next chapter, "A Brief History of Popular Diets," he gives some excellent background on diets in general. One point he makes — one that most diet books skip over — has to do with the political components of diet research. Here he also does a good job of covering what he calls, "Fat versus Carbs: The Great Debate." He refers to the work of Harvard's Dr. Walter C. Willett and what he has written regarding fiber. (We will be taking a look at Willett's book a bit later. His work shows that if people have plenty of high fiber in their diet the danger posed by most fats becomes minimal.)

Then it's on to the Glycemic Index. He tells how in the late 1970s Dr. David Jenkins at the University of Toronto introduced the concept of the Glycemic Index. In his research he found that eating certain starches such as white bread or white potatoes increases blood sugar levels faster than table sugar. This Glycemic Index concept is a hot topic now when it comes to understanding how the body stores fat. Almost any new diet book is going have to take it into account.

In the next section called "Understanding Popular Diets," he discusses different diets and gives a nice thumbnail sketch of their problems without being snippy. In fact, he even has some nice things to say about Atkins! But he adds that the big problem he has with the Atkins plan is saturated fat, and he gives detailed reasons why. After Atkins, he then moves on to Dr. Dean Ornish's diet program. He says that it is similar to Pritikin's and has some of the same drawbacks, which he says Ornish acknowledges, and that is because it is difficult to follow. (We will look at both of these plans later on.) He concludes this section with a nice flourish saying that he knows and admires both men and recognizes their fight against the established order to help people with weight and health problems.

Starting with a section (he doesn't number chapters) called "A Day in the Life," he gets down to specifics, starting with a stress on eating a good breakfast. As he goes on discussing what to eat, he gets to lunch where he says, "Don't even think about limiting the amount you eat," which has got to sound fantastic to anyone who has tried a low-calorie diet. He stresses forgetting about calorie count, fat grams, or portion sizes. In mid-afternoon you can have fifteen almonds or cashews (which sounds like "counting" to me.) Then on to a dinner of fish, lean meat, etc., finishing with a low- or no- carb dessert.

The next section, "Good Fats, Bad Fats," gives a good examination of trans fats, triglycerides, and cholesterol. His discussion of LDL particle size is well worth reading and isn't found in most diet books.

In the next part, "Hello, Bread," he suggests starting to add more high-fiber carbs, which he says that you should do "gradually and attentively." About here he seems to get onto some rather muddled ground. For example he says to watch the addition of carbs and cut back if you stop losing weight. But then he states, "I'm not talking about weighing yourself every day. I'm actually opposed to that." He then adds that you can usually tell when you're putting on weight, and if you can't, your clothes will let you know. Maybe you are a person with a talking wardrobe, but I've found that by the time my pants start to get tight then the diet is dead. To me this is one of the big weaknesses of this plan. It is true, particularly for women, that body weight will fluctuate on a monthly basis, but you need a better indicator than what he suggests.

I'll skip on now to his suggestions and observations on certain foods. For example, one interesting point he makes that I have never found elsewhere is that sourdough is better for you than most white breads because its acidic quality decreases its Glycemic Index. In"It's Not Just What You Eat, It's How You Eat It," he makes several good points. The one that struck me the most, and I think should be included in any good diet book, is the simple statement "in every vegetable or fruit, the younger when picked, the lower the carb count." Later in this section he gives another good tip I haven't seen elsewhere. He says you can lower the Glycemic Index of any meal if 15 minutes before eating, you have a spoonful of Metamucil in a glass of water. This slows down the meal's absorption.

In the "How Eating Makes You Hungry" section, he reports on a study done by Dr. David S. Ludwig, which showed that when the highly-refined-carb breakfast is compared with a "South Beach" type breakfast, the latter does a much better job of preventing hunger longer. Also in this section he gives a good thumbnail list of foods and their Glycemic Index. Look this over. I think you'll find some surprises as to which foods are the high and low ones.

When it comes to exercise, I think he is mistaken. He wants exercise to be "something you can incorporate easily into your routine." I can't help but feel that is part of what got you into the condition you're in now. The "easy answers" to exercise is the most common kind of poor information on the subject found in diet books. He claims that you have achieved your goal when you break a sweat and that 20 minutes is plenty.

When it comes to supplements he says he takes aspirin, fish oil, and a statin drug. He says you should take into consideration the fact that most cardiologists he knows over the age of 40 take a statin drug even with no sign of heart problems. He says that the cost is around $3,000 a year. Maybe this is a good plan; the research seems to look encouraging.

But two things come to mind: Most medical doctors I've known seem to be pretty quick to go for a pill. Also, they have the income (or get freebies from the drug companies) to afford this practice.

The last two-thirds of this diet book, like most others, consists mostly of meal plans and recipes.

THE PALEOLITHIC PRESCRIPTION

S. Boyd Eaton, M.D., Marjorie Shostak, and Melvin Konner, M.D.,Ph.D.

This next book takes a much more historical look at the diet question. Although it is now over twenty years old, it is well worth a look for several reasons. First, although it surely wasn't the first to take a "cave man" look at diet, it was the most popular and one of the best reasoned. Also the authors had the university degrees and positions to give weight to their statements. At the time this book was written, S. Boyd Eaton was a medical doctor and Associate Professor at Emory University School of Medicine, Marjorie Shostak was Assistant Professor of Anthropology at Emory, and Melvin Konner held both M.D. and Ph.D. degrees and was a professor of anthropology at the same school.

They start by pointing out, as others have before them, that we are pretty much the same people genetically as the hunter- gatherers of old. We have many advantages they did not, but when it came to many modern illnesses, for them these illnesses were either very rare or simply didn't exist in their world. They died mainly from infections, complications of child birth, or trauma. Not us. We're too clever for that. Instead we die mostly from diseases that we build ourselves. The authors give as an example how, before 1940, Native American Indians had almost no diabetes and now, only some seventy years later, it's prevalent. Teeth found from Cro-Magnons and Paleolithic humans had almost no dental cavities. And when they did occur they were small. Most of us are walking examples of a pretty big change.

So why did these hunter-gatherers lose out to the farmers? The authors say it was just sheer numbers. As game got more scarce, farming produced both more people and food than the hunters. So here we are only a few thousand years later with SUVs and arthritis, belly-button rings and heart disease, air conditioning, and diabetes. I'm not knocking it. Not many of us would trade our supermarkets and air conditioning for a cave and a sharp stick. But I think that all of us could do without the diseases. And these writers think that is possible.

To show how rapid and drastic this change has been, they point out that there were more than 100,000 generations of hunter-gatherers, 500 generations of farmers, and a little more than 10 generations of ourselves that have lived in the industrial age. They compare the diets of these groups, and we don't win.

This difference in diet shows up in several ways. For example the authors have good evidence from anthropological digs to show that Mediterranean hunter-gatherers 30,000 years ago had an estimated height of 5' 10" for males and 5' 6" for females. Also examination of these remains shows they were not only larger but also more robust than the farmers that followed them.

The authors then make a telling comparison of physical evolution and cultural evolution. The first is a slow process controlled by populations and physical environmental conditions. But cultural evolution can accelerate much faster. Weapons, tools, and farming technology can develop at a rapid pace. Society was fairly stable for thousands of generations. With agriculture this change started to accelerate. And then came the Industrial Revolution. Change, drastic change, took place in only 200 years. And that included a big change in diet as well.

On pages 47 and 48, the authors make a point that is the main reason that I chose to review this book. To me, this is a major piece of information that you would think would be more widespread. It is this: Heart attacks and strokes, to a large degree, are caused by a buildup of plaque in the arteries.

Now here's the fact that I found very surprising: From autopsies of young men killed in World War II, Korea, and Vietnam as well as those killed in auto accidents, it was found that even healthy young people in their teens and twenties had already started to line their arteries with plaque! Compare this with a study of the bodies of even middle-aged men from what they call pre-industrial societies (Arctic tribes, Solomon Islanders, etc.), which showed no signs of this condition. Of course, they stress that this is due to diet.

They then go into a lengthy description of the diet of hunter-gatherers. And here we find another bit of information that you can't help but wish had gotten more publicity. Today's meat from domesticated, feed-lot animals is 25% to 30% fat on the average. Compare this to wild game meat that is about 4% fat. This increase of fat makes the domestic meat much more tender and juicy. But the big difference is that this juicy, tasty fat also has a different chemical composition than the fat from wild game. Wild game has a far higher proportion of polyunsaturated fatty acids. In fact, it has as average of five times as much as the same amount of supermarket beef. Wild game also contains about 2.5% of eicosapentaenoic acid which they say is a heart-healthy addition. Domestic beef? Sorry, almost none.

And the other big change was the one you hear more about — dietary fiber. Much more fiber back then, much less now. Along with this came that other wonderful product that we all unfortunately love — sugar. About the only real sweetener in the Stone Age was honey, and this was a great rarity. Today sweeteners of all types provide around 20% of all caloric intake in the modern diet.

This difference in nutritional content doesn't stop with meat but exists in most of our other foods as well. The authors make a good comparison of the plant food then and now. At the end of this chapter they give a detailed comparison of the Stone Age diet and our own. Some examples: they ate about half the fat and three times the protein. The fat that they did eat was more of the polyunsaturated type. Their carbs were, of course, all unrefined. Also, and here is probably another important point, their salt intake was about a quarter of ours. And they consumed much more potassium than sodium as well as twice as much calcium. And the list goes on.

In the next chapter, the authors keep expanding on the changes in diet and the possible effects. For example, the wheat, potatoes, and corn we eat today weren't around just a few thousand years ago. But all three are often a major part of our diet today. They say that even this would not be such a big problem if our current diet provided the same ratios and quality as before. Again they go into great detail as to the "what and whys"of this. How dramatic this change has been, starting a few thousand years ago and accelerating in the last two hundred, is covered in depth.

Before we leave this book I would like to pull out one other nugget that many diet books also stress. They point out the following: We are designed by evolution to overeat. And not just overeat but eat as much fat as we can get our hands on. This makes good sense. For thousands of years you were never sure when or where the next meal was coming from, so when you got a chance you ate — and you ate a lot. Twenty thousand years ago there were not a lot of young women around saying, "Oh, no more for me, I'm already up to a size two!" This "overeating" was a big advantage when you might go a week or more between meals. But that problem of missing meals is long gone.

That about covers the high points of this excellent book. I do wish these authors would do an update. A lot has been learned about diet in the last twenty-five years that could impact some of their ideas.

THE PALEO DIET

Loren Cordain, Ph.D.

Well, as long as we are wandering around with the Stone Age crowd, let's look at another book that takes a similar approach. Published some fifteen years after the previous title, this author adds some information that is worth having. On the first page of the introduction he points out that we are still genetically the same as old Igor with his stone ax. He then goes on to say, "Many of our health problems today are the direct result of what we do — and do not — eat." Yes, that sounds familiar because most writers in this field say pretty much the same thing. He also stresses the same things that we have heard elsewhere, among them that these ancestors were much healthier than we are prone to assume.

Right from the start, on page ten, he tells us what these people ate and what they didn't: No dairy, almost no cereal grains, no salt except what was already in their food; the only sweet was honey; animal flesh dominated; the only carbs (plants and fruit) were unrefined and the major fat was mono- or poly-unsaturated. Pretty much the same eating plan that we keep hearing about.

However, he is not a fan of the Atkins type low-carb diet because he thinks it lacks enough fruits and veggies and includes far too much saturated fat. His mantra is again what we keep reading — saturated fat bad, monounsturated fat good. However, he is a long way from the anti-meat crowd. He says that lean meat will help you lose weight as well as slow your appetite. It was nice to see that he quotes some good research that shows that there is no harm to the kidneys from a high-meat diet as has been claimed by other diet gurus. In fact, he recommends four times as much protein as you find in the average diet. On page 21, he lists his specific diet recommendations: Eat lots of lean meat, fresh vegetables, and fruit. Then, in his "Seven Keys of the Paleo Diet," he makes a point that I haven't run across very often. He suggests eating a diet with a "net alkaline load."

He hits this acid-alkaline balance idea several times in the book. On page 52, he gives a more complete description of why he thinks this is important and says, "Very few people — including nutritionists and dietitians — are aware that the acid-base content of your food can affect your health." He comes back to this point again and again, even including, on page 213, a detailed list of the acid-base values of common foods. I can't comment one way or the other on this acid-base idea, but I do know that this is the only place I've seen it stressed the way he does.

He says that you cannot overeat on the Paleo Diet. Overeating, he believes, comes from an intake of some combination of sugar, starch, fat, and salt in highly concentrated forms. He says that when any of these foods exist in nature they carry with them nutritional components like fiber, vitamins, and minerals. He then states: "The notion that humans were meant to be vegetarians runs contrary to every shred of evolutionary evidence from the fossil and anthropological record." He says if we had been vegetarians we would have ended up pretty much like our nearest animal relatives, the chimpanzees. Chimps are mostly vegetarians and they, like the gorillas, have the large bellies needed to extract the food value needed from this type of diet.

In explaining our ancestor's drive for big-game hunting he gives a good example of how it takes energy to kill either a mouse or a deer. But your pay-back with the deer is much greater, and that is why early man learned to hunt larger and larger animals. But, he adds, they couldn't just eat lean meat because they would suffer from "rabbit starvation," a term, he says, describes a condition caused by eating only meat. To prevent this, he says, they needed to eat carbohydrates, and that's another reason he's hot for carbs. I think that he could be wrong here. This condition was first discussed by Stefansson in his book *My Life With The Eskimo* written about 1912. He said it was caused not by just eating meat but by not getting enough fat in the diet.

A bit later in the book Cordain gets to the section called "Hello Grains, Hello Health Problems." And here is one of the big reasons I wanted to include this book. He goes on at length as to how this change, from hunter-gatherer to farmer, brought with it many of today's health ills. We got shorter and weaker; we developed arthritis, diabetes, heart attacks, and other problems. And then the changes kept on coming. Around 200 years ago the Industrial Revolution brought refined sugar, canned foods, refined white flour, and much more. Then, in the 1950s, research started to point to the connection between eating meat, butter, etc, and heart attacks and colon cancer. The researchers blamed meat, but we know now that the real problem probably centered around mixing refined carbs and saturated fat. But back then the call went out, "Don't eat meat." Cordain doesn't point this out, but this was the start of the "no-fat" craze that is proving to be such a disaster.

A few pages later he says. "One of the great dietary myths in the Western world is that whole grains and legumes are healthful." He goes on to say that these foods, when it comes to good nutrition, are marginal at best. Compounding the problem was the addition of hydrogenated oils, sugars, and other sweeteners. By the 1970s, industry had developed high-fructose corn syrup which saved the food-processing companies money over using sugar. This product may slam the body harder in regard to insulin production than even old-fashioned sugar, which means more weight gain and a faster road to other problems. He points out that there are about ten teaspoons of high-fructose corn syrup in a twelve-ounce can of soda. Also, our annual average consumption is about 83 pounds of high-fructose corn syrup and 66 pounds of sugar. And those number are increasing year by year.

On page 64, Cordain gives a good explanation of why all calories are not the same. For example the body burns 12%

more energy digesting protein than it does carbs. And this, coupled with the better appetite satisfaction from proteins, is why, he says, it can produce weight loss.

He ends the book by giving examples of what to eat and what not to eat, followed by that old diet book standby — meal suggestions and recipes. But he also includes something that I've only found in his book and that is a list of companies where you can buy wild game meat and fowl.

I wish that he would update this book because he has some interesting ideas.

NEANDER-THIN: A Caveman's Guide to Nutrition

Raymond V. Audette with Troy Gilchrist

As long as we are examining the caveman connection, this is the next logical book. The title of this book could just as well be *Eat Raw,* because that's a big part of Audette's advice. Unlike the writers of most diet books, the author wasn't motivated by a desire to lose weight but by his deteriorating health. By age 34 he was suffering from both rheumatoid arthritis and diabetes. He had gotten to the point where he could only work part-time and things looked pretty much downhill. That's when he started his research. He found, as had many before him, that his ailments were "diseases of civilization." Hunter-gatherers didn't have these problems.

Farmers did. He, of course, was not the first to make this observation but he adds an interesting note. He claims that from skeletal remains it can be shown that "arthritis followed corn as it made its way from Mexico to the rest of the world."

So he decided to go back to the hunter-gatherer life style and eat only food that would be available if he was, "naked of all technology save that of a convenient sharp stick or stone." Then he writes, without any apparent attempt at irony, "Armed only with the sharp stick of my criteria I headed for the supermarket."

After eating this way for a while, his health started to improve, so he headed to the library to see if he had developed something new. He found that this type of diet went back as far as the 1790s. He then spends several pages covering what he calls immune-system disorders caused by diet. Also, he finds that all of these same problems are also caused by obesity.

Like many other diet-book writers, he points out that restricted-calorie diets don't work in the long run. He also lists another fact that I have found elsewhere: "Overweight people usually eat significantly less than people of normal weight." As others have also pointed out, he says the low-fat craze has been shown to fail (he quotes the studies) on several counts.

On page 16, he hits another point that you are seeing more often in newer diet books. And that is that we are a primate with a single-chambered stomach. That means that, unlike animals with multi-chambered stomachs, we are not equipped to do a good job of digesting many of the carbohydrates found in nature. He makes an interesting observation. Most primates live in tropical forest or at its edges. This is because that is the environment that provides the fruits, vegetables, insects, and small game they need for food.

He also points out that we are the only primate that has all of the following: A big brain, bipedalism, a lack of fur, and a unique variety of sweat glands. This combination of physical characteristics gives us the capacity to kill and eat a larger variety of animals than any other species. He then spends the next several pages showing how each trait has lent itself to our success as a species. His take on this is the big reason that I included this book. Few other diet books give it this much coverage, and I think it's important if you are going to understand the reasons behind the most effective diets.

After several pages of conjecture about how we went from hunter-gathering to farming, he says that over time we developed the technologies that made it possible for us to eat foods like grain, dried beans, potatoes, milk, and refined sugar. And it was then, he believes, that the nutritional deficiencies hit the biological fan. For example, we are the only animal that continues to use milk and milk products, not from ourselves but from other animals, long past infancy.

On pages 44-45, he lays out his "Ten Commandments" of what to eat and what not to eat. It's about what you would expect with some interesting exceptions such as peanuts and chocolate as well as turnips and yogurt on the "Do Not Eat" side. On the "Eat" side are also some eye catchers like bananas, mangoes, and pineapples.

About his only suggestion on exercise is his recommendation to increase physical activity. He says that the best kind of exercise is the kind where you "do not have to change your clothes." He goes a bit further when he gets to the end of the book where he has included a "Frequently Asked Questions" chapter. To the question "Should I exercise more?," his answer is, "Yes, but only in moderation." Then rather surprisingly he adds, "Strenuous exercise has more risks than benefits and should be avoided." I find it strange that many of the older writers in this field seem to be clueless when it comes to exercise.

In addition to the question-and-answer portion, he also throws in some recipes and menu suggestions. As I've mentioned before, to fluff out a diet book almost all authors do this.

In the very last paragraph of the book on page 66, before getting into questions and answers, menus and recipes, he gives a dire warning: If you start this plan and then quit you will "gain weight faster than ever before." Also any cheating on the diet will "immediately result in illness." I can't help but feel that this dire warning is more than a little bit overblown.

DINE OUT AND LOSE WEIGHT

Michel Montignac

The big reason I've included this book is that it is the only diet book I've read over the last 50 years that includes a seven-page list of which wine to drink for any given illness! Acidosis? Drink Fumé Blanc. Asthma? Drink Grey Riesling or Barbera. For bloating, drink Champagne. And the list goes on. He also has a lot of good things to say about chocolate. So it's safe to say that this is a "different" diet book. As you may have guessed, Montignac is French, and this book was first published in France in 1987. Several years later it was translated into English and published in the United States. His book will move us from the caveman condition to white linen and good silver.

When he wrote this book, Mr. Montignac was an executive with a large pharmaceutical company in France. The title comes from the fact that in this position he was often called upon to entertain visiting dignitaries. In this role he found himself gaining weight and started a great deal of research to see what he could do about changing that. He came up with a way that a person could do all of this entertaining and still lose or maintain a desired weight. He notes that aside from Japan, France has the lowest average weight of all the industrialized nations. He sees this changing as American fast-food choices arrive, and so another reason for his writing this book was to warn his countrymen not to lose their traditional eating habits.

Starting with Chapter Two he goes into a rather technical description of the Glycemic Index. Remember, this was written over 20 years ago, and not many diet books had picked up on this idea. He also points out that processing increases the index of any food. For example corn has an index of 70, but corm flakes have one of 85. On page 37, he talks about something else that was very new wave at the time: "good" and "bad" carbohydrates. Next he gets to fats. His is about the standard take on saturated, unsaturated, and polyunsaturated fatty acids. He does say that it is his opinion that the popular view of saturated fat being all bad is a bit of an over-reaction. Then on to fiber. His is about the standard opinion here also. He ends the chapter with a list of good and bad carbs.

Chapter Three has an eye-catching opening sentence: "The calorie theory is probably the greatest scientific swindle of the twentieth century." He tells how this all got started by the research done by Newburgh and Johnston at the University of Michigan in 1930, which was published in *The New England Journal of Medicine*. Four years later the same publication published serious reservations about these findings, but it had already been taken up as gospel. Mr. Montignac does a good job of showing why this whole calorie thing is pretty much a guessing game.

His take on fruit is interesting. On page 96 he says, "Fruit is a taboo subject, and I know that if I dared ask you to eliminate it from your diet, you would probably close the book immediately." His hard-and-fast rule: "Fruit must always be eaten alone!" He also suggests that you should always eat fruit on an empty stomach. He says to eat it first thing in the morning and then wait at least 20 minutes before eating a carbohydrate breakfast. Another option is to eat fruit three hours after a meal. I keep running across similar suggestions from other diet-book authors. Given that "fruits and vegetables" seems to be the opening lines of most diet suggestions, this always looks a bit strange. He then goes on to provide a detailed list of what foods to eat and when to eat them. As do many other diet book authors, he makes a point of saying that you should not skip meals.

After "Phase I," which is the weight loss phase, it on to "Phase II," which is a life-long eating plan. As he outlines this plan on page 169, he makes a statement that I don't think is quite true. He says, "Man is the only living animal that eats combined foods." I don't think that he has spent much time on a ranch or farm. It's been my experience that both pigs and chickens will eat about anything, combined or otherwise.

If you have any doubt that this book was written by a Frenchman, just turn to Chapter Eleven. This is the chapter on wines. As he tells it, wine is good for just about everything. No, you can't drink it during Phase I (the weight-loss phase), which he assures you he is very sorry about. Also you can't drink wine on an empty stomach, even in Phase II. But outside of that, get out the corkscrew! He points out that his grandmother hated water, only drank red wine, and she lived to be 102 years old.

And if that wasn't French enough, how about Chapter Twelve: "The Marvels of Chocolate." He is quick to point out that he is not talking about some cheap candy bar, but high-quality chocolate with at least 60% cocoa or higher. Yes, he likes chocolate, but back in Chapter Ten, "Sugar is Poison," he goes on at length about this evil food but then fails to mention that it is a large component of any chocolate treat.

I think that in Chapter Thirteen he is just plain wrong. The chapter's title is "Exercise Does Not Cause Weight Loss." Again, maybe this is the French attitude of 20 years ago on the subject. As you read his examples, you get the feeling that his only approved exercise is lifting a case of Bordeaux.

He ends the book with a "Technical Appendix" listing all of the data behind his eating plan. The big reason I included this book (in addition to the wine and chocolate) was that it was one of the first that I read that gives a hard-and-fast rule on eating only carbohydrates at one meal and proteins and fats at another. Like many later diet books, he takes a "kind of" Atkins approach. I say "kind of" because Atkins is a full-on proteins-and-fats diet with almost no carbs at first. Montignac's plan is that you can eat both but not together.

THE ZONE

Berry Sears, Ph.D. with Bill Lawren

With this book we start to move more toward the middle ground in the "Meat vs. Plants" diets.

The big attention-getter in this book, for me at least, was the way he starts the first paragraph of the preface. He says he's a walking genetic time bomb. His grandfather, father, and every one of his three uncles died of heart attacks before the age of 54. As he wrote this he was forty-seven. I would have gone to the nearest bar — he went to the library.

My guess is that Sears may have done more research on the subject than any other author I quote. But it's still the same basic mix of excellent information, good information, and some questionable information that we have seen elsewhere. Let me make one minor complaint to start: If his editor had just told him that he could use the term "The Zone" only 50 times in the entire book it would have gone a long way in improving his writing style. He whips this phrase to the point you began to feel he's selling a product, not an idea.

Also in the preface he describes the hormone Eicosanoids, saying it is a cornerstone of his system. There are hundreds of these hormones, and they became the basis of his research. He tells us that his book is all about using food to manipulate an Eicosanoids balance. And this is a passport to— you guessed it— the Zone. (Yes, he always capitalizes the word.)

By page seven he is taking on some of the big boys of the diet field by stating that the low-fat, low-protein, high-carbohydrate diet of recent popularity was way off base. He adds, "Much of the current wisdom is dead wrong." He points out on page nine, in the chapter called "The Fattening of America," how and why this happened. He feels it was caused by the poor information that we were given by scientists, nutritionists, and the federal government. This was to eat less fat and more carbs. It wasn't working when he wrote this book, and by now the no-fat, high-carb mantra has been pretty well discredited.

He says that to get a new perspective on food here's what you need to know: Eating fat doesn't make you fat, excess carbs do. It's hard to lose weight by restricting calories. Diets based on choice restrictions and calorie limits usually fail. Weight loss has little to do with will power. (A lot of diet books make this claim. I'm afraid that I have my doubts on this point.) Food can be good or bad. And finally, the biochemical effects of food have been constant for the last forty million years. He ends this list of statements by saying that the bottom line is just a matter of reaching (you guessed it!) the Zone. He goes on to say that nutrition, like religion, is extremely visceral. And finally, weight gain or loss is not the goal — the objective is to lose fat.

Then in the section "Carbohydrates — The Reason You're Fat," he gives a full description of how high-carb diets get you fat and how little it takes. In explaining this he gets to our old friend the Glycemic Index. One statement he makes regarding the index is that, because the sweetener in fruit is fructose, fruit has a very low Glycemic Index compared to other sweeteners. Remember this was written some fifteen years ago and I'm not sure that statement has held up. He does follow it with one that I think is still safe. He says taking the fiber out of fruit and only drinking the juice makes the index soar. He says that fat and protein are the two bad guys of nutrition mythology. Again, look at the time frame. At the time that he was writing this, that was all too true.

Next he gets to the section called "Protein — The Neglected Macronutrient." He says the practice of regarding all fats and proteins as bad was a case of throwing out the baby with the bath water. He then gives a long description of why the low-carb, high-protein diet is wrong. I'm not sure that Sears would take the same approach today. Here, however, he claims that this type of diet causes a permanent change in fat cells in the body making weight loss harder over time. He also takes the standard line that ketones are bad guys and should be avoided.

Then he gets to what he calls the Fat Phobia. Here he makes a statement that would probably be regarded as even more true today. "What's the most feared three-letter word in the American dietary dictionary? F-A-T." And he says that this fat phobia is at its worst in the United States, and yet nowhere else in the world are people so fat. But when it comes to eating fat, it is his strong belief that you have to eat some fat to lose weight.

When he gets to Chapter Three, "The Hormonal Effects of Food," he hits full stride. Hormones are his area of study, and he goes into a great deal of depth as to how this all works. He stresses that "Food is the most powerful drug you will ever encounter." And learning how to use it is your passport to, once again, the Zone. Also, he admits that there are people who can eat potato chips, pasta, and ice cream and never gain weight. The reason for this , he says, depends on your genes.

In Chapter Four called, "Eicosanoids — The Short Course," the course is not all that short. Should you have a burning desire to cover the subject in depth, as he does, since this is his area of study, this is the place. I'll just take his word for most of it. But this chapter does show what I think is a weakness in his approach. Because he is so deeply involved in the study of the process that he describes, it all seems quite obvious to him. But it gets a bit too complicated for the average reader.

His suggestions in Chapter Six, "Exercise in the Zone," are about what you would expect. He gives a full description of not just the "what" but also the "why" of how the body reacts to different kinds of aerobic and anaerobic workouts. He adds that a high-carbohydrate diet may interfere with your exercise goals. To get the maximum benefit you must keep in (cue the trumpets) the Zone.

In Chapter Seven, "Boundaries of the Zone," he gets down to exactly how to eat to get the Zone effect. He says that every time you eat you should achieve a certain balance. This involves getting a three-to-four ratio between proteins and carbs. He goes on to say that this ratio may vary to some degree depending on the genetic makeup of the individual. If you are one of the lucky ones, which includes about 25% of the population, who have a low insulin response to carbs, you can get away with eating a bit more carbohydrate. One nice point he makes is that the general guidelines on protein are of doubtful value because this need varies from person to person.

That is why, I guess, he sticks to ratios rather than specific amounts. He doesn't talk about fat here. In a pie chart for the Zone diet on page 71, he does show a ratio of 40% carbs, 30% protein, and 30% fat. But the focus of this chapter is the protein-carb balance.

It's not until the next chapter where he goes into great detail about "balancing" your meals that he gets to fats. There he finally makes the "good fat-bad fat" distinction that we are used to seeing. The bad fat is of course saturated fat. And the villain here is the arachidonic acid in saturated fat which is the building block for bad eicosanoids. He says that you should restrict — if not eliminate — these from your diet. He says that foods high in this acid are egg yolks, organ meats, deli meats and fatty red meat. The good fats, as I'm sure you have already guessed, are the monounsturated ones. Later in the book, as he discusses these foods and their ratios, he says that the diet of Stone Age man had the same combination and amounts that he prescribes in the Zone diet. He says his source for this statement is to be found in an article in a 1985 edition of the *New England Journal of Medicine*. I didn't look up that article, but I think this statement sounds a bit off.

Next he gets into man's move from hunting to farming and he says that this introduced two new food groups — grains and dairy products. Remember that this was written over fifteen years ago when whole-wheat anything was king.

He then adds, "by and large humankind has been genetically unable to cope with these foods." Milk is an interesting example. All humans are born with an enzyme that can break down the lactose in milk. Most people lose this enzyme by the time they reach adulthood and so have trouble digesting milk or many milk products. Scandinavians are one group that keep that enzyme throughout their lives. Why? Evolution. The same with grains. These are high-density carbs and most of us aren't programmed for them. The way he covers this problem is one of the big reasons I like this book.

From here on he covers vitamins and minerals and how they work in our bodies. In Chapter Twelve he gets back to his favorite — Eicosanoids. And this goes on for pages. Again, some of it gets a little complicated, but he does make a good, easy-to-understand point on page 131: "But remember: the best amount of supplementation is always the least amount." He then goes on to discuss at some length high blood pressure and high cholesterol. Before you take medication for these conditions, I strongly suggest you read this section. Then on to a long discussion of chronic diseases and how he feels that diet can help them. He makes the point that this is not a "diet to lose weight" book, but a "diet for good health" book.

I think that this book has two big problems: The first is that this is a very complex explanation of how food functions in the human body. It is so complicated that, unless you are very dedicated and like detailed explanations, you may give up some hundred pages in. The second problem comes from his eating plan itself. It is pretty complicated to follow. I'm not saying it's bad or wrong, but I'm not sure that the average reader would be able to stick to this plan over the long haul. He has done a great deal of research and it is worth your time to read it if you do decide to go in this direction.

THE PRITIKIN PROGRAM FOR DIET AND EXERCISE

Nathan Pritikin

Let's jump over to the other side of the "Eat my way or die" debate. If you really want to have dietary twitches, just go back and forth, as I have for years, trying to come up with some middle ground in the great diet wars. I've pretty much come to the conclusion that there isn't much in the way of consensus. So let's leave the "kill it and eat it" believers and go and listen to some of the "roots and berries" crowd.

The hard-line believers in this group are the full-on vegetarians or vegans. I have some friends in the vegetarian camp who are happy and healthy with their choice. There can be a bit of confusion between a vegetarian and a vegan. The vegetarian belief has a long history and in some cases has religious roots. The vegan belief seems to be much more extreme, in that vegans not only believe in a plant-based diet but also reject all other animal products. It is probably expressing my bias to say that the vegetarians have strong feelings about what they should eat, whereas the vegans have a strong belief about what everybody should eat.

I'm going to start our stroll down this agricultural lane with a book a bit less than a full-scale vegetarian agenda. The book is *The Pritikin Program for Diet and Exercise*. It might seem strange that I would pick a book that was published 30 years ago, but I picked it because it has some excellent points to make that still hold up today. I'm sure there have been changes in this program over time but I think it was his reputation and success that moved many of his beliefs into the mainstream.

Published in 1979, his plan had been around for some time before that. And this was no small-time strip-mall operation, as shown by his client list, which included people like George Harrison, Gloria Swanson, Candice Bergan, Issac Bashevis Singer, Bill Walton, and others. He starts out by saying that all fats, both animal and vegetable, are hazardous to your health. He then moves on to what he describes as "the world's healthiest diet." On the first page of chapter one he tells us that his diet "is low in fat, cholesterol, protein and highly refined carbohydrates, such as sugars." Now that he's got our mouths watering, he says that his diet is "high in starches, as part of complex, mostly unrefined carbohydrates, and are basically foods as grown, eaten raw or cooked." He makes no bones about his love of carbohydrates which he calls the best food you can eat. But he then points out that he is not a complete vegetarian but advises limiting meat of any kind to four ounces a day. He adds that if you can reduce that amount to three time a week, so much the better.

He follows this with a very complete table of foods to eat and foods to avoid, which is about what you would expect: Egg whites, but only seven a week, but only two if raw (he doesn't say why the difference), but no egg yolks. Only cheese with 1% or less of fat by weight. Here is a bit of a strange one: all beans and peas are fine with the exception of soybeans. Perhaps soybeans have too much protein for his liking. And no nuts except chestnuts. They are probably OK because of their low fat content. All vegetables except avocados and olives are allowed.

I found this interesting: He recommends bread, cereals, crackers, rice, pasta, tortillas, baked goods, and other grain products — but here is what struck me as a bit strange — as long as they are made without fats, oils, sugars or egg yolk. And, of course, to round it off, no alcohol or caffeine.

Up to now I've been a bit dismissive of this plan, but it is only fair to point out again that this book was written 30 years ago and I'm sure there have be some changes along the way. And here's the bigger point: I've known several people that have gone on this plan, and all lost weight — in some cases a lot of weight. And those who could stick to the plan with a bit of tweaking here and there kept the weight off and enjoyed good health while doing so.

Back to the book. One thing that caught my attention was that on page 25 he gives a brief description of the Tarahumara Indian tribe in Mexico and their diet. His book is one of the first places in which I ran across a reference to this tribe outside of anthropological studies. (Later, in my own section of the book, you'll hear more about them).

In the section of his book called "What Carbohydrates Do," he gives what is still today a good description of what "bad" (sugars, honey, etc.) and "good" carbohydrates do in the body. Any hard-core vegetarian could use this ammunition.

In Chapter Seven, he gives the basic principles of his plan. He says that every day you should eat a couple of kinds of whole grains, a raw vegetable salad, raw or cooked green or yellow vegetables, a piece of citrus and three or four other fruits. Then he adds beans or peas three times a week if you like them, once a week if you don't. Also sweet potatoes or hard yellow squash once or twice a week. Then for vitamin B12 he says you should eat six ounces of low-fat, low-cholesterol animal protein per week. There are other minor suggestions, but I thought it was interesting that his instructions include the stress of eating three full meals a day and snacks if you feel hungry between meals. This last part was a bit ahead of its time.

Now we get to Chapter Twelve. From there through Chapter Fourteen is the big thing I would brag about regarding this book. And that is the way he stresses exercise! Back when this book first came out, if you tried to jog in most cities, people would call out to ask what was wrong because they were sure there must be a problem. I have a friend who started jogging in Denver about this time and was stopped by a police officer who asked if there was a problem. It seemed that people had called in about him running. Pritikin uses the term isotonic (dynamic) exercise. He gives as an example walking and running. This is today's aerobic exercise. He describes isometrics exercise (today's resistance exercise) and gives weight lifting as an example. But the point is, he stresses it where other popular diet books of the time don't even mention it. How much exercise does he suggest? He says one-half to one hour twice a day! Walking briskly is good but jogging is better. He says to start out slowly and work your way up.

His take on exercise is the big reason that I included this book. Others before him had suggested it. One that comes to mind is Jack LaLanne. But LaLanne was too often looked upon as just another "health nut" and very few in the medical industry gave him much notice. That "health nut" LaLanne lived into his nineties. And where almost all of the diet experts now recommend exercise, most of them don't give it a lot of space and say things like "20 minutes is enough" or "just walk until you start to sweat." Pritikin said flat out that it was a necessary part of any plan for good health.

I think it's safe to say that Pritikin, in many ways, was far ahead of his time. I believe that today this plan would add some things (fish oil, etc.), but you can see how he was a stand-out when he started his program.

DR. DEAN ORNISH'S PROGRAM FOR REVERSING HEART DISEASE

Dr. Dean Ornish

With this program for reversing heart disease we look at a different kind of diet book. This is pretty much a strict vegetarian approach. It's true that in his later writings he started to add some oils, chicken, and fish to the diet, but not when he first started.

On the cover Dr. Ornish tells us that this is "The Only System Scientifically Proven to Reverse Heart Disease Without Drugs or Surgery." This statement alone sets this book apart from other standard diet books. This is more of a "Fix your heart, get healthy, get in touch with the inner you, and maybe drop a few pounds while you're at it" type of book. Although aimed at heart patients, its greater success was as a good-health and weight-loss guide. If you look at the acknowledgments at the first of the book you can't help but be just a bit stunned at the number of names. To say that he thanks over 200 people wouldn't be an exaggeration. This seems a bit much.

On to the book itself. I think he would be quick to point out, and he's right, that he didn't plan to write a diet book but a book for heart patients. But I'm going to include this book anyway because he has some interesting ideas regarding diet. For one thing he's not a "my way or the highway" type of doctor. For example, on page two he says "our program need not be all or nothing," but he does feel that if you have severe heart disease you should stick to what he calls the "Opening Your Heart" program. He says that this is a different type of procedure, one based on love, knowledge, and compassion. He goes on to talk about healing "not only the heart but the soul." OK, look, I should point out that this is way too much touchy-feely, love beads, and patchouli oil for my taste. Having said that, I should add that I can guarantee that if I ever have a major heart problem you will probably be able to find me in the lotus position, chanting my mantra and chugging down tofu. But for now I'm afraid I have never been a great fan of soul repair. But about the time that you start to get a bit tired of all the "New Age" attitude, he gets you back on his side with a statement like the one on page 27. There he says that when a patient comes in with severe chest pains asking someone to get the elephant off his chest, "I don't just feed him broccoli and ask him to start meditating."

He goes on to make a statement that is one of the reasons I wanted to include this book. This statement is "the third-party system of reimbursement (health insurance, Medicare, etc.) encourages the use of drugs and surgery rather than health education." Then on the next page he says something that I've found nowhere else. He opens by pointing out that doctors often set the best (or worst?) example of this approach. They have learned to separate themselves emotionally from their patients. To emphasize how destructive this can be he points out the following: As a profession, doctors have among the highest rates of drug addiction and divorce of any identifiable group. Also the average physician dies ten years prematurely, and doctors' suicide rate is one of the highest. And he says that it is this emotional separation that makes them hold their focus on drugs and surgery.

I mention the above because it all too often applies to the medical profession's approach to diet, and not just the lose-weight diet but complete nutrition. But to be fair, physicians have more than a full-time job just trying to treat full-blown illnesses. The vast majority of the time, when the average patient shows up, the damage of poor diet has already been done. Given the complexity of modern medicine, it's about all a doctor can do to keep up with the illness parade let alone specializing in healthy diets.

Ornish takes a dim view of many of the current approaches to treating heart disease. If you do have any kind of heart disorder, read his take on bypass surgery as well as angioplasty. You can see why he headed off in another direction. When it comes to the root causes of heart disease, he says that lifestyle factors are the major villains. Although he doesn't say so, this same thing could apply to diet and overall good health. He also says that diet, exercise, and quitting smoking are important but also feels it's important to quiet down your mind, listen to others' feelings, and to your own, and finally "to give and receive love more fully." (Wow!)

When it comes to exercise, he's not a big fan. On page 73 he takes a cheap shot at Jim Foxx, the man who wrote a good book on jogging. Ornish uses this as an example of how people can die from vigorous exercise. Foxx himself pointed out that he held off his death by jogging because he knew he had a genetic heart problem. It's true that Ornish is writing for heart patients, but still his take on exercise doesn't sound right.

Another reason that I included this book is the suggestions he makes in Chapter Five. It's here that he talks about his meeting with Swami Satchidananda and this man's influence on his life. I'm not a great fan of Eastern religions, but there are parts of these beliefs that are worth a look. Although usually referred to in Western culture as religion, it is really more of a system of suggestions about behavior. What you might want to ask here is "what does this have to do with diet?" Good question. The point that he makes is that "mind set" is important to your well-being, and my point is that this very same thing affects diet.

On to his eating ideas. His plan, in another book published in 1990, has changed quite a bit, but his main points probably remain about the same. On page 255 he tells you how bad all fats are for you. His "reversal diet," as he calls it, is pretty much strict vegetarian. He says that his diet is not designed to restrict calories, but then he goes to some length to show how research studies (and he lists them) find that animals on reduced-calorie diets live longer and are healthier. Unlike many people espousing vegetarian diets, he allows a bit of alcohol and moderate use of salt and sugar. But he is hard and fast on the "no-meat" rule. In fact, he's not only anti-meat but pretty much anti-animal protein in any form, saying he believes it can cause health problems.(Note: When we look at his next book you will see how he backtracks on this.) In this book he, like other vegetarians, says that you don't need animal protein to be healthy and lists the foods that, if eaten in the right combinations, will meet the same protein needs. He claims that this combination of foods is exactly the same protein that's found in steak. I'm no chemist, and I know that this belief is popular with this group, but I question that assertion.

On page 261 he gets a bit carried away, listing the health problems that can be expected by not being a full-on vegetarian. He is even against olive oil! Remember, this is a "heart healthy" book, and he claims that any oil in your food will increase cholesterol levels.(This attitude changes in some of his later writings where he recommends a bit of fish.) Finally, he goes all out and says, "Many anthropologists believe that our ancestors were primarily vegetarians." What? I would like to see the names of these anthropologists. I think it's only fair to suggest that they not quit their day job at the drive thru.

Salt. After all of his hard-core vegetarian rant, I was surprised that he's not all that worked up about salt, considering that this is a book aimed at heart patients. He simply says that unless a person is salt-sensitive, salt shouldn't be a problem.

And now we get to exercise. Yes, this book is older, but his attitude here still parallels too much of today's standard medical approach to exercise. Take his statement: "The good news is that you don't really have to exercise very much in order to get most of the health benefits." He uses the research done at the Institute of Aerobics Research to imply that "walking 30 minutes a day reduces premature death almost as much as running 30 to 40 miles a week." But his own charts, and he gives them to substantiate this, show that in men, the difference was 25.5 deaths per 10,000 for the walkers and 18.6 for the runners. Now I'm no math whiz, but isn't that around a 25% difference? And with women the difference was even greater! But he says this is not significant. Then he spends some time warning that there is a chance of a heart attack with vigorous exercise. It was pretty well established, even back when this book was written, that the danger increases a great deal more with no exercise.

Let me add one closing note. I'll admit in advance that I've taken some cheap shots. This book was written over 15 years ago, and people are bound to change some of their ideas, considering all of the advances in this field. In an issue of *Newsweek* magazine, Ornish wrote a guest column where he makes many of the same points that he does in this book — with one glaring exception. In the next-to-the-last paragraph, where he is talking about what to eat, he tells us how we should eat the good old standbys like fruits, vegetables, whole grains, legumes, soy products "and some fish." But somehow, I just don't think that his heart was in that last part.

THE SPECTRUM

Dean Ornish, M.D.

This is Ornish's latest work, which hit the bookshelves in early 2008. An earlier book, *Eat More, Weigh Less*, was more of a standard diet book, but this comes closer to a revision of his earlier book that we looked at above. As I mentioned in the first review, in some of Ornish's more recent writings that he did for popular magazines, he began to include a little fish and chicken in his suggestions. This also shows up in this new book.

The very first sentence of this book starts "I just had a piece of chocolate." But he quickly adds that he is not cheating on his diet but "enjoying" his diet. And then the reason for the title: He is going to give you a "broad spectrum" of choices when it comes to diet. He also assures you that he "used the latest in high-tech, expensive, state-of-the-art measures" to prove his points. And he goes on to tell how the research done by his group has been in collaboration with the most credible scientific investigators at major academic medical centers. He then lists some 17 medical journals where his work has appeared as well as medical textbooks. And this not too subtle self-aggrandizement goes on for some time. But it is for a reason: He wants you to know that his is one of the most scientifically documented alternative medicine approaches around. And this I believe to be one of the main reasons that his approach has enjoyed an increasing popularity over the years. He is probably as sincere and dedicated as anyone in the alternative-medicine field today. There are problems but these will be listed at the end of this review.

You can tell he is more than a bit tired of his approach being called radical. He asks how radical is his approach compared to having your chest sawed open for a bypass operation. If you can improve your health without stents, angioplasty, or other physical invasion of the body, he feels it makes sense to try. And here, I believe, is the strength of his approach. Yes, he may go a bit overboard on the touchy-feely part, but much of his argument makes sense. And he has a great deal of documentation to back it up. It is also his strong belief that the health care industry is not paying enough attention to the prevention side of the health equation and is instead spending huge amounts only "after the fact." He asks if it is radical to "ask people to walk, meditate, quit smoking, and eat fruits and vegetables" if this can be shown to be a real help in many cases.

He quotes a Canadian study called INTERHEART (yes, it is always capitalized; I don't know why) that followed 30,000 men and women in 52 countries on six continents, which found that factors related to nutrition and lifestyle accounted for 95% of the risk of heart attack. But, he says, very little money, compared to the cost of treating heart diseases, goes to prevention. We are starting to see more of the mainstream medical groups go in this direction. Maybe not as much of the "meditation and group hug" approach but at least much more of a "stop it before it happens" with proper diet and exercise.

All that being said, Ornish still, on occasion, has a tendency to go a bit too far out on the ethereal plane. When in Chapter Two, "Why It Works," he lists the ten reasons, number ten is "The most powerful motivating force in the universe is love," which might give some people pause. Also number four is "How you eat is as important as what you eat." I'm not sure that is 100% true for many of us. Number six, "It's important to address the deeper issues that underlie our behaviors." It is true that you see more and more psychologists and psychiatrists publishing in the field of diet, and for the truly obese there may be good reasons. But it is my own feeling that this approach can easily be overdone. Since many of the points he makes in this book are similar to the ones he makes in the book we have already examined, let's look at two specific points that show a real change from the first book.

The first would be fats. Yes, he, like most others, opposes saturated and trans fats, but his take on some of the others is not as mainstream. In his first book he is not at all fond of Omega-3 from fish oil. On page 279 in that book he tells us why he recommends getting your Omega-3s from plant sources. But in this new book on page 43 he says, "I've been taking fish oil for many years and have been advising just about everyone else to do the same." What!? As science advances and new information is acquired, it is to be expected that people will change their minds. But if they are good at what they do, you expect them to explain how and why this change happened. His handling of this makes one doubt some of his other findings.

I think that what it comes down to is that, despite all of the positive results in new research on fats, Ornish still has a hard time pulling up his vegetarian roots. Although he may suggest a little fish or chicken it still is pretty much 98% veggies. Also, at a maximum of 10% fat in any of his suggested diets, he still believes in a much lower percentage of fat than almost all of the other major players.

The other change, which is not as dramatic as the fat approach but is worth mentioning, is his take on exercise. He does a much better job this time and his suggestions are more mainstream and more detailed.

I believe that Ornish is still at heart a vegetarian and also there is always a strong whiff of Eastern Philosophy in many of his ideas. I'm not claiming that's wrong, but I think this makes him a bit less objective in some cases than you might hope. Also, he is simply disingenuous when he goes to some length in his first book to tell all of the problems with fish oil and then in this book he says he has used it for years and recommended it to others. The same thing is true regarding exercise. He is almost dismissive regarding exercise in his first book but lauds its virtues now. We all change our minds but when those changes are as pronounced as the ones here, it would seem to require a fuller explanation.

EATING WELL FOR OPTIMUM HEALTH

Andrew Weil, M.D.

Dr. Weil is a hot name in the health and diet world not because he has come up with some big new scientific breakthrough but I think at least in part, because he must have a top notch publicist and/or agent. Like Atkins, Sears, Dr. Phil, and others he's as much an industry as he is a health guru. He has churned out ten books and numerous booklets, a health letter, CDs, and two online web sites, as well as fronting for a supplement company, a line of cosmetics, and even a dog food brand. An issue of *Nutrition Action Health Letter*, a publication of the Center for Science in the Public Interest, points out that he makes around two million dollars a year from all of this. He claims that all profits go to his foundation. But when Nutrition Action checked the 2003 and 2004 tax returns for the Weil

Foundation, it showed them receiving nothing.

I'm not criticizing the man for trying to make money, but it does make me a little uneasy to take his suggestions on products that are going to make him a dollar. Now, all of that being said, I still found some very good information in his book, *Eating Well for Optimum Health*, published in 2000, the book we'll look at next.

On the first page of the first chapter he points out how the American Council on Science and Health suggested ten resolutions for a healthy new year. He says that it includes the standard suggestions of don't smoke, etc., but only one brief suggestion on diet. It suggests that you eat a balanced and varied diet as well as avoiding obesity and fad diets. It then goes on to add that there are no good or bad foods. His comment: "I find this advice to be remarkably unhelpful." He goes on to ask, "Eat a balanced diet? What is that?" Then he talks about some foods that sure sound good or bad to him.

Regarding diet and disease, he makes an interesting point on page 21. During World War II when people in Denmark, Holland, and other occupied areas were unable to get foods high in saturated fats (butter, cheese, etc.), the rate of heart attacks dropped. After the war, when they could get these foods again, the rate went back up. Also Japanese women have one of the lowest breast cancer rates in the world. But when they come over to this country and adopt our diet, the numbers rise. He goes on to give other examples of diet affecting disease. But then we get to the part where he starts to show a mild inclination towards self-aggrandizement.

For example he writes glowingly about a herbalist in Singapore who works out of an excellent restaurant. He tells this local healer that he has no appetite and is constantly cold. The herbalist checks the pulse of his right hand, looks at his tongue and says he's too "yin." His prescription: An order of baked lamb with Chinese wolfberries and a pot of double-boiled chicken soup. These being "yang" dishes, they should fix him right up. This advice is of little use to most people because they won't find wolfberries or double-boiled chicken soup at their neighborhood market, but this is an example of his not too subtle way of exhibiting his extensive travels and research.

So why does Weil take this approach? I think that one of the big reasons is that he has a very good understanding of his customer base. The people he's pitching to are mostly the baby boomer crowd, a great many of whom have for years been the primary customers for the Alternative Medicine, Eastern Philosophy, etc. approach. They grew out of the long-hair and tie-dye age and having reached their Birkenstock and Volvo years, they are starting to have to deal with the wrinkles and sag of deep middle age. Wanting to turn into anything but their parents, they keep looking for the magic potion, ointment, or diet that will keep them "cool." Weil is a very bright, sensitive super-salesman, and he knows how to reach this group and does it better than anyone in the diet industry today.

At the start of Chapter Two he tells how two types of diets have become popular in the last 30 years: low or no-fat and low-carb. He covers the diets of Ornish, Pritikin, Montignac, Atkins, and Sears. He then asks if you want a "plant-based" diet or a "carnivorous free-for-all?" From that last statement you get a feel for where he falls on the issue. He then moves on to compare the no-fat, low-carb, and all-veggie schools. He tells us that there are disagreements and no one has all of the answers, but he stands tall, asks for a touch of backlighting and bravely states, "I am not afraid to speculate or to try to make good guesses as I venture into unknown territory." (Music up, move to close up.) He then assures us that he will "always base my speculations on the best available scientific evidence as well as common sense." Wow! I kind of guessed that's what everybody in this field thought they were doing.

Next he comes up with some reasons why a no-fat diet could be unhealthy. The problem is the lack of essential fatty acids, especially omega 3s. He knocks Ornish for his low-fat approach as well as Atkins for his ketosis theory. He says proteins have their own problems. And, of course, saturated fats are the bad guys.

Around page 50, where he is talking about the dietary habits of Stone Age people, he makes a strange comment. "Few individuals lived beyond what is now considered youth." I'm not sure where he gets his data for this statement. Most of the anthropological reports on grave sites of pre-agricultural societies don't support this. There will be more on this in some of the other books we will look into because it does tie into diet.

He then goes into a good explanation of the Glycemic Index. He was one of the first well-known authorities in the field to give such a detailed description of this index and what it means, not just for weight loss but also for general good health. Also, it is here that he makes a point about wheat flour that, I think, will be noted more and more in the future. He points out that bread, all bread, is in the high glycemic range not just because of its nutritional content but due to mechanical reasons. The milling of grain breaks it down into fine particles and the leavening action of yeast further increases the surface area. He agrees with others that whole wheat is much better for you because of the nutrients it contains, not because of its Glycemic Index. He goes on to give a good and complete explanation. I think that he gets carried away with this when he criticizes Sears, Atkins, and Montignac for all lumping bread and pasta in the same category. He claims they shouldn't do this because "scientists have clearly established that pasta has a much lower Glycemic Index than most breads." I haven't run across this "clearly established" fact anywhere else.

I was startled to read that he does not think that table sugar is all that bad for you. This is the only diet book that I've read that even comes close to giving that opinion. He feels that the problem comes when sugar is paired with other foods. He ends his pitch for sugar with one of his not uncommon statements that exemplifies the rather strange observations that he comes up with from time to time that are pure Weil: "If you want to evolve toward living on cosmic energy instead of gross material food, you should probably start by eating more sugar, as that is the food closest to the source." (What!?)

After the above bit of weirdness he comes back down from his ethereal plane to give some excellent advice regarding flour. He feels that this finely ground product may well be a major contributor to our nation's epidemic of overweight and heart disease. I think that he deserves a great deal of credit for being out in front with this opinion. More experts in the field are coming around to something close to this judgment on flour and flour products. Keep in mind that anyone who takes this position is going up against some very large organizations like agribusiness and the processed products companies, as well as the Federal Government. I think that this is one of the most important observations that he makes. And he follows it up with a statement that is part of the same line of reasoning. The big problem, he feels, is modern technology and its refining and processing of low glycemic foods into high ones. He gives the example of flour and corn syrup. A number of authors agree with him on this, but he gives one of the best descriptions of how and why it happened. After a couple of pages fleshing out the above ideas he ends up by saying that he thinks that 25% to 30% of the general public is very sensitive to the effects of these carbohydrates.

As we move on we get to the part where he slams the low-carb diets, saying that he thinks that most of the weight loss is water loss. He goes on to suggest that if they keep losing weight it is probably that the diet is so boring that they just eat less. He even goes so far as to say that a low-carb diet "may" break down muscle tissue. And that statement just "may" be one big stretch. Next he again gets a bit "new age" when describing this type of diet, he says, "Moreover, it removes from the diet foods that establish cultural identity, reinforce social connection, and provide satisfaction as well as sustenance."

On to part three of Chapter Two where he gives you his take on fats. By now this has become more mainstream but when he first started writing, this take on the subject wasn't that popular. He gives a long, excellent description of the different kinds of fats and how our bodies process them, including omega 3s and omega 6s and why we need both for good health. He follows this description with a statement that seems to make good sense. The ratio of omega 6s to omega 3s in the modern diet is out of balance. He goes to some length to explain why he feels this is so. His final point here I found particularly interesting. After he explains why he feels this is a problem, he says that this imbalance, more than what we eat, may explain many of today's health problems.

He, like most others in the field, is a fan of olive oil. And here is one of the things that is so intriguing about Weil. About the time you've had it with his twilight zone stuff he comes up with a statement that makes you stop and think. This is true regarding his observation of olive oil. He says the reason that olive oil is so different is that other oils are extracted by heat or high pressure or both. But olives, being soft, make it possible to extract the oil much more easily. Also olive oil has the highest percentage of monounsaturated fat of any edible oil — a good reason for its popularity.

From there on you get a high-powered sales pitch for semi-vegetarianism. Oh, maybe a little free range chicken or wild fish, but basically it's vegetarian. Many of his comments on diet would seem to be open to question. However, he does come down on the side of the Mediterranean Diet as proposed by Dr. Walter Willett whose book we will look at later.

I'm convinced that Dr Weil is slightly overweight. No, I can't prove that, but if you look at the back-combed beard to hide the chubby cheeks and the full-cut shirt worn with the shirt tail out to hide a bit of a gut, it sure seems to point that way. And look at page 179. He spends the whole page and part of the next pointing out how overweight isn't really all that unhealthy. (This same idea hit the news awhile back and was pretty much exposed as wrong.) As far as his suggestions as to how to lose weight? He says to count calories and control hunger. Not exactly a new concept.

As we get to the end of this book he slips in another ethereal bit of information. He says "I also want to discuss a topic I consider important that nutritionists, dietitians and doctors never mention: The spiritual quality of food." (No, these people don't mention this because it is a religious not a scientific premise, and most people in these fields consider themselves scientists, not spiritualists.) He goes on to discuss the spiritual quality of food and its "vital energy." He also says to take into account the "emotional and spiritual vibrations of the people who have handled it."

And finally, on the same point, look at Appendix D, on page 278, entitled, "The Possibility of Surviving Without Eating." I won't go into great detail here but anyone who plans to follow his suggestion on healthy eating might want to get a copy of this book and read these three pages for themselves because I'll just cover it briefly. In this section he tells about a Qigong master named Yan Xin. Weil tells us that, "The fact that his disciples are mostly doctors, researchers, engineers, and other well-educated people, many of them working in the West, makes their stories of having not eaten for months or years more compelling and accessible." This state is called "Bigu," he says, and goes on to tell us how the followers, "almost all with M.D. or Ph.D. after their names," give glowing accounts of this. He ends by saying, "Please bear in mind that I am simply reporting secondhand information," but you get the very strong feeling that he buys it.

I have a very big problem with all of this. Here is a man that is on a medical school faculty, writes for *Time* magazine as a health authority, and is often seen on various television network shows. You have to wonder, have the people that hire him read his stuff? I think that over the years he has modified or even abandoned some of his more outrageous pronouncements, but it still gives the reader pause. But he also does have some good, practical ideas that are worth considering.

HEALTHY AGING

Andrew Weil, M.D.

Before we move on, let's take a quick look at one of Weil's latest books, *Healthy Aging,* published in 2005. As I've pointed out before, Weil is very sensitive to his market, which I guess to be people in their 40s and 50s, and this book is aimed at that group. Also, I think that someone — maybe his agent, publicist, or publisher — got him to tone down many of his over-the-top suggestions.

As usual, he has some good advice. He says that he doesn't look at age as a reversible process so the best approach is to go into these natural changes as healthily as possible because common sense tells us that aging is a fact. This, of course, is true, but I have known people who, in middle age, decided to change. They started to eat wisely and exercise, and a couple of years later, they sure looked a lot younger.

When it comes to ensuring a longer, healthier life, he turns to the findings of The MacArthur Foundation Study of Aging in America. This well-respected study points out that of all the different groups studied, the one thing common to all people who seemed to know the secret of aging well was that they all were physically active all through their lives and maintained social and intellectual activity. Yes, there were the groups that ate only vegetables and those that didn't, the yogurt enthusiasts, the meat eaters and so on, but it was the above factors that always showed up at the finish line.

In this book, like many of the other newest diet tomes, he actually had a good word to say about Dr. Atkins. Weil admits that Atkins was the one who should get credit for pointing out the role of carbohydrates in obesity. From there he goes into the standard "good carbs bad carbs" discussion. Some of this is a bit of a new take on some of his earlier writings.

Also, about here he shows that he has not completely given up his wing-nut side. After giving a good description of how to age gracefully, he then tells us how he chased tornadoes for two weeks in Texas. Oh, and "This past summer I ran with the bulls" in Pamplona, Spain. On the other hand, as a concession to aging, he has backed off backpacking. Maybe it's just me, but I would still choose backpacking any day over the chance of getting trampled by a bull. Of his own diet he says, "I have not eaten meat in more than thirty years, being a pesco-lacto-vegetarian." Isn't that diet definition just bit pretentious no matter how specific it might be?

Then on to Chapter Eleven, which deals with physical activity. He starts out with his, by now, standard pitch on how overweight isn't all that bad. As I've mentioned before, I think the good doctor is a bit plump himself, and this fact seems to push him to make some pretty questionable statements when he tries to support the concept of being "husky." But starting around page 182 he gives some great recommendations on how to exercise, including suggestions on the type of exercise, equipment, and duration.

From there to the end of the book he gives advice on relaxation and stress reduction that contains a lot of good suggestions. He makes the point that you can practice breathing exercises and meditation without any association with religion. Now and then, Weil shows a good sense of humor. For example he gives a clever parody of the old advice that has become the Serenity Prayer that starts off, "God, grant me the serenity." The parody that he quotes goes, "God, grant me the senility to forget the people I never liked anyway, the good fortune to run into the ones I do, and the eyesight to tell the difference."

All in all, this is one of his best books. He gets off track now and then but it is still worth a look.

THE ULTIMATE WEIGHT SOLUTION

Dr. Phil McGraw

At last we come to a diet book that to me is a disaster. It is included because it resembles far too many of the other standard diet books written today. Yes, there are a few good parts, but in the main it fails for the same reason that most of the hundreds of others that you can find on the shelves of any large bookstore fail. For this reason, I'll give it more coverage than it deserves. Most of these books are written for women who can turn to Dr. Phil's show so they can get some kind of pleasure from the problems of others. And this, and many other diet books, are aimed at this market by telling them something to the effect of, "Here is the easy way to change your life. Oh, and your problems aren't your fault!" Reading the three-and-a-half pages of acknowledgments, you have to be impressed. But, of course, that is what they're for. You'll notice they don't say that these people all endorsed the book, just that they were of help. The one person whom he thanks who should have been at the head of the list is his agent, Jan Miller. My guess is that she only had to point out that the two big areas of book sales were diet books and cookbooks and, not wanting to miss any good bets, he wrote both!

And so, on to Phil McGraw's advice on diet. He tells us on page four that "I have to get totally real with you." He then warns us that his plan is not going to be a quick fix, but if you do what he tells you on every page of this book, "Nothing will stop you from being anything other than healthy, vibrant, in shape and fully in charge of yourself and everything you think, do, and feel." But then this firm father figure warns you that he's not going to tell you just what you want to hear. But not to worry, he is going to tell you the truth. Does it bother you when someone keeps telling you how they are going to be "totally real" and stress that they are going to tell you the "complete truth" as well? It does me.

Then on page nine he gets down to the Dr. Phil nitty-gritty with his "The Seven Keys to Permanent Weight Loss." You probably guessed that it starts off with "Right Thinking" and "Healing Feelings." Oh, and one of the "keys" is

"Intentional Exercise." Probably some good tips here as I'm sure you, like me, often accidentally do sit-ups. All right, there are some good ideas in his "keys" but to me, it seems like there is also way too much smoke.

Moving on, he says there will be no calorie counting or memorizing of exhaustive food lists. In fact, he assures you, you are going to learn about food in a completely different way. A way that no one or no diet book has ever done before! And it gets better. On page 17 we get to a section entitled "You Don't Need Willpower." And here is his ground-breaking news: You have been lied to by the diet industry when they tell you that you need willpower to control your weight. Then our good Dr. Phil "liberates" you with the news that you no longer have to rely on willpower because it doesn't work. But then two pages later he points out that "it may be hard at first." Doesn't that sound to you that it might take just a smidgen of willpower at that point? I know this sounds like nitpicking, but much of this book seems to take the approach that if you just invent a slick new word, you've accomplished something real. As I'm sure you have guessed by now, I do not agree.

But there is no point in discussing this book if all I'm going to do is take cheap shots, so let's take a look at the page where he gives a good, honest table of suggested body weight. For women who are seriously overweight this gives them some realistic goals. He also tells you how to measure to get your waist-to-hip ratio. You're going to hear more about this ratio in diet and health publications.

Then we come to the section called "Set Your Goals." You can guess how much it hurts me to have to admit that this section is excellent. In fact, it is a good program for almost anything you really want to accomplish. When we get to "Your Readiness Profile," which is a list of 20 questions, I can assure you that if you can answer "yes" to all twenty and you're telling the truth, you could not only lose weight but also become rich, successful, happy, and anything else you might want. But the point he is trying to make is a good one. And that is if you want something, and I mean really want it, then a full-scale commitment is the answer.

After that brief brush with reality, we move on to another test where you can rate your "Weight Locus of Control." Wait, that's just the overall term. Included are tests for "Internal Weight Locus of Control" as well as, and I'm sure you guessed this one, "External Weight Locus of Control." And that old favorite, "Chance Weight Locus of Control." All of this leads you into things like an "Internal Dialogue Audit" and how to "Maximize Your Weight Loss Through Self-Talk." Then it's on to "Externalizing/Internalizing" as well as "Labeling" and "Frustrating Thinking" and much more. My personal favorite — "Catastrophizing."

Of course it doesn't end there. No, you find out how to "Analyze and Respond to Your Self-Talk." You even get a table for that. From there you get to things like how to "Gain Emotional Closure" as well as a "Personal Environment Audit." No, it doesn't involve global warming.

At long last on page 190 we get to his diet plan. Its pretty much the standard low-fat, whole grain, etc. you would expect. But when you get to his meal planning you have to wonder if he did any research at all on nutrition. For example, the first suggested dinner includes a sirloin steak and a baked potato. From there it's pretty much of a flashback to the diets of the 1950s.

But he does have one section that is good and in some ways better than you find in the average diet book — and that is his section on exercise. Yes, there is some of his standard jargon, but many of the ideas themselves are good, and he takes a much more sensible approach than some. He says that if you are out of shape, start off gently and gradually and build up a little at a time. Table 8 on page 224 gives an eight-week plan that moves you along at a pace that almost anyone can follow.

But enough about the numerous problem books on the subject. Let's move on to a book that despite my moaning about some minor points, is one of the better books in the field.

THE OMNIVORE'S DILEMMA

Michael Pollan

Let me start with two things about this book. One, it is not a standard diet book. And two, at times I will complain about his writing style. So why is it here? Because the writer does a lot of excellent research that we need to examine. And when it comes to his writing style, the fact is, he is a much better writer than I am, so there could be traces of jealousy or it could have more to do with my age, what with my being old and all. The style he uses is the popular one where you spend a lot of time making sure that your reader knows that you are sensitive, ethereal, caring, etc.. For example, when he is going to go hunting for a wild pig, we get page after page about his emotional reactions to the whole thing. After a while you just want to say, "Just shoot the damn pig!" At last he finally does, but it nearly gives him a case of the vapors. This is a popular style both for the "with it" literati as well as some of the academic crowd.

But despite all of my complaints, this doesn't really matter because what we want to look at is his take on the way food of all kinds goes from hoof or field to you. Also his research on processed food itself is well worth reading. So, all my sniping aside, let's get to the book. (After my taking some cheap shots at his writing style, this review is followed by one of his next books, *In Defense of Food*, in which he drops any whiff of pretension and writes an excellent book as we shall see. But back to this one.)

His basic plan is to follow the food chain from hoof or field and look at the different ways it is done and what this can mean to you, the consumer. Early on he quotes the English author William Ralph Inge who said, "The whole of nature is a conjugation of the verb to eat, in the active and passive." And Pollan does an excellent job of doing just that, following the food chain, better than anything else I've read. For example, take plain old corn. Do you have any idea how much corn you eat and in what different forms? How about modified starch, unmodified starch, ascorbic acid, lecithin, dextrose, lactic acid, lysine, maltose, high-fructose corn syrup, MSG, polyols, caramel coloring, and xanthan gum? All from corn.

Next we get to the part that is the primary reason I'll use this book for reference later. He has the writing skill to make things like a feed lot, a slaughterhouse, or corn processing not just interesting but easy to read about as well. I use the term "feed lot," but as he points out, they are now called CAFO — Confined Animal Feeding Operations. And they are gigantic! Seventy or eighty years ago, it took around five years to raise a steer to slaughter size. In the 1950s this changed to around two or three years. Today it's fourteen to sixteen months. The way they made this happen was by penning the steers up and feeding them corn, about 32 pounds per animal per day. Along with corn come other grains as well as things like animal fats, protein supplements, antibiotics, liquid vitamins, synthetic estrogen, and a bit of alfalfa and silage. Because this is not their natural diet, there is a real problem with illness. That is just one reason why 70% of the antibiotics sold in the United States goes to agribusiness. You would think that the thousands of tons of cow manure that this produces would be a good source of fertilizer. No, it's too rich in nitrogen and phosphorus as well as heavy metals and hormone residue. I think that by now you have a pretty good idea that the steak you had this weekend wasn't quite the product you thought it was.

Another subject that he does a good job of covering involves sweeteners. Like a lot of things our consumption of them has increased with time. Consider that four hundred years ago about the only sweetener available to the average family was honey and consumption averaged less than a pound a year per person. He points out that by 1985 this was up to 128 pounds per person of all kinds of sweeteners, and by now it is up to over 158 pounds per person and still increasing. Also, it's in a lot more products, and most of it is high-fructose corn syrup.

Pollan quotes a statement by an English agronomist, made some years back, to the effect that when it comes to good health we should consider the whole system — soil, plant, animal and man. That still sounds like good advice. Along that line Pollan looks at the organic movement. He points out that there is a struggle between what he calls "big organic" and the original organic movement. He gives a good description of how "organic" has gone mainstream and what all of that really means. Also his description of the difference in fat content and character of grass-fed and pen-raised animals is well worth reading.

Pollan is a good researcher, so keep an eye out for articles he writes in popular publications. I respect what he is trying to bring to our attention. He is one of several of the authors that I have reviewed who do this.

IN DEFENSE OF FOOD

Michael Pollan

Remember how I whined about some aspects of this author's writing style in my review of the previous book? Well, you won't find it in this excellent little book. Pollan, like many of us, is getting tired of raging conflicts over different diets and how minuscule differences are whipped up into mountains. He points out that foods have, for centuries, changed a bit from one generation to another but today the changes are accelerating at what he calls a dizzying pace.

He points out that much of this is the product of a thirty-two-billion-dollar food-marketing machine that pushes for change because it means more products to sell. He also notes that the constantly shifting ground of nutritional science doesn't help. He says, "Sooner or later, everything solid we've been told about the links between our diet and our health seems to get blown away in the gust of the most recent study." He shows how the sacrosanct low fat-diet that was supposed to help prevent cancer and heart disease didn't stand up to scrutiny. Also fiber may not be the answer for colorectal cancer, and fish may or may not, due to mercury content, be all that great for some people.

How all of this got so complicated, he says, tells us a lot about the institutional imperatives of the food industry, nutritional science, and his own field, journalism. For all of these groups, the idea that for hundreds of generations we had done a pretty good job of eating without supervision couldn't be turned to their profit. And so, Pollan says, "like a large gray cloud, a great Conspiracy of Scientific Complexity has gathered around the simplest questions of nutrition — much to the advantage of everyone involved." And from there he does an excellent job of describing and dispersing that large gray cloud.

He certainly doesn't mean to imply that there isn't a problem. He believes, as do many others, that the "Western diet," as it is often called, has produced a number of the "Western diseases" like obesity, diabetes, cardiovascular diseases, and several kinds of cancer. I know that this term is a popular way to describe the type of diet common to much of the modern world. But this seems to imply that it is only found in Western societies, which is not as true today as it was at one time. What it refers to today, more than perhaps anything else, is processed or mass-produced foods.

Pollan uses the term "nutritionism," which is a word that he says was first coined by an Australian sociologist, to describe the popular focus of those involved in selling, producing, and studying food. He makes a point of saying that this focus is on using information about the content of different elements in food to make claims and pronouncements that will advance careers and sell products. There should be no confusion between nutrition, a scientific term, and nutritionism, an ideology. He feels that this shift from eating foods to eating nutrients had its greatest push in 1977 by the report produced by the United States Senate Select Committee on Nutrition and Human Needs. Other writers also list this as an important watershed event in the diet wars.

It's true that this may have set a national direction for diet, but as he points out, as far back as the 1950s a belief called "the lipid hypothesis" was coming into vogue. This hypothesis held that the consumption of fat from meat, dietary cholesterol, and dairy products was the culprit regarding "Western diseases." The American Heart Association was one of the first to embrace this belief, but many others, despite the lack of a great deal of hard evidence, were quick to follow.

But it didn't stop there. The results of this Senate Committee's inquiry at first started to list specific foods in their eating suggestions but this ran into conflict with some big Washington lobbies that represented these products. And so the politicians and their staffs started down the road to "nutritionism." By using scientific euphemisms and jargon and bringing in nutrients, they were able to escape the wrath of the major players. Pollan gives an excellent example of how this worked. To show the power of the sugar lobby, he points out that the Senate report listed the maximum amount of sugar permitted in the daily diet as a whopping 25% of all calories! And to show that their power hasn't diminished, when the World Health Organization recommended that no more than 10% of calories should come from sugar, the lobbyists had a political fit. Through aggressive lobbying they worked to get this changed, even threatening to pressure Congress to cut off funding to the organization.

Nutritionism has produced some rather strange results. Pollan gives the example of margarine, the first important synthetic food to become a diet staple. It started as a cheap substitute for butter. Then along came the lipid hypothesis.

The margarine makers figured out a way to remove cholesterol and saturated fat, which they replaced with "good" polyunsaturated fats and about any vitamin that was wanted. This was fine, and sold well, until along came a problem, and with it a new buzz word, "trans fat." That was a problem because that's what margarine was. But, no worries, because the whole thing is an artificial product; it was no great feat just to do some re-engineering. And so today it's trans-fat free. And you will never see it advertised as imitation butter, even if that is what it is. Why? Because the manufacturers don't have to. They may have at one time because there used to be a law requiring this. But the food industry did a good job of heavy lobbying to change the law that used to require that designation. And, of course, they won.

This was no small victory and surprisingly enough they were helped, he says, by groups like the American Heart Association. Why? Well, by this time the AHA was deep into the "fat wars," and they were eager to get people off saturated fat and on to vegetable oils. Back then this included vegetable oils such as margarine, which at the time was trans fat. In fact, the AHA called for the modification of many foods to remove saturated fats and cholesterol. For this reason they pushed Congress to remove any restrictions on the marketing of these modified products. And of course the food industry was more than happy to help. And this meant there were a lot of very profitable semi-foods to be manufactured and sold.

The great problem I have found in doing these reviews is that when I find an excellent book, like this one, I go on far too long. So let me just suggest that you add this to your reading list.

This need for reference books becomes more and more important as we, at long last, start to get some reliable information about diet and good health.

CANCER: DISEASE OF CIVILIZATION?

Vilhjalmur Stefansson

Now let's take a quick look at a much older book that looks at diet in a different way. I wanted to include it because Stefansson is a person I admired because of his dedication to researching the human condition on all levels. This book was published in 1960 and got little attention at the time.

His purpose in writing this book was to show that people who had not been touched by what we call modern civilization but still lived and, more importantly, ate as they had for centuries had very little or none of the many diseases that we have in modern society. For much of his information he goes back to the records and writings of people who lived with, or frequently visited, these groups. People like missionaries, ship captains, federally-appointed doctors, and others who kept records. His own experience in the far north, over a number of years, was the source of his early interest in this subject. He quotes at some length the findings of these people and how they all reported a lack of diseases like cancer, heart disease, diabetes, arthritis, and tooth decay among the native people. Equally impressive, a number of these writers were able to report on what happened to these same people as they started to adopt the eating and living habits of outsiders, who began to visit them more and more. The results were not positive.

Something else that he mentions was how the discoveries of people like Pasteur and his germ theory and the work of others in the cell structure of disease had a downside that is never acknowledged. He says the problem was minor compared to the great medical advantages of their work, but what it did was shift the attention away from carefully reporting over long periods on things like the diet and living conditions of different groups and how it affected their health. I mention this because a lot of years later we are starting to go back to this type of research as shown in things like the Harvard Nurses' Study and others. No, not an exact parallel, but in many ways similar.

Another nice thing about this book is that he shows the even-handed approach of the true researcher. Having spent years in the north and adopting their eating habits (he himself ate meat almost exclusively for the rest of his life), you might expect him to stop there. Instead, he then looked for groups that took the opposite approach and lived mostly on a vegetarian diet. He found them in northern India in the state of Hunza. Several people had done detailed studies of this isolated group that ate almost no meat. Stefansson then points out that he thinks that this shows there is not just one way to good health through only one kind of diet. But there are certain conditions that seem to hold true: Food with very little or no processing, regular physical activity even into old age, and close relationships in an extended family.

The following has little to do with diet, but if you want to get a good inside look at what field research was like around the turn of the last century find a copy of Stefansson's earlier work called *My Life With the Eskimo*, published in 1912. His description of almost starving and other experiences are told without a lot of attention to how they deeply affected his psyche or how they cramped his karma.

THE DIABETES DIET

Dr. Richard K. Bernstein

This is not anything like the standard diet book. Instead of a "lose a few pounds" guide, it's a "Try to stay alive" book, which means that the author isn't casual about his ideas. Keep in mind that he writes his books for diabetics.

These are people who, if they continue to eat poorly, don't just get fat, they die. This minor fact makes them a bit more attentive to what they eat than the rest of us. And because what they eat is so vital to their health, we can pick up some useful tips from their food choices. Also it's worth noting that this is a disease that is increasing rapidly and much of the reason for this, Dr. Bernstein and many others feel, is diet.

Dr. Bernstein, himself a diabetic, says in the book's very first paragraph, "Indeed, I can make a claim that no other diet author can — that my own diet saved my life." (Yes, I know, Dr. Sears said something along the same line, but Bernstein has a better argument.) Bernstein has had diabetes from an early age, and although he followed all of the standard prescriptions, his health kept getting worse. And that is why he went to great lengths to study the disease. Most other diet books are written based on observation or experience with patients or lab work, and a lot of good work has been done. But I can't help but believe that when it's you who feels like you're dying, you just can't help but try a little harder.

He started out, around 50 years ago, on the typical low-fat, high-carb diet that was the standard treatment for diabetes at that time. But he kept having problems. Then he went on a low-carb diet without any fat restrictions, and that is when things turned around for him.

He didn't come out of college as a physician but as an engineer. However, as his health got worse, he spent more and more time researching his problem. He found some research that had been done with animals that he thought looked promising. Using this as a guide, he went on the same type of low-carb diet and had good results. And about here we get to the action that he took that I think deserves real admiration. Seeing that this plan worked so well for his problems, he tried to publish his findings. But he tried to no avail because he wasn't a member of the medical fraternity. And here is what I find so impressive: If they wouldn't listen to an outsider, he decided he would become an insider. So at the age of 45 he walked away from his engineering career and went to medical school.

When he started his own practice he found that most diabetics that came to him for treatment were Type Two diabetics, not Type One like himself. Whereas he had fought to gain weight, they couldn't lose it. He tried the same diet plan and found that whereas it had helped him gain, it helped them lose weight. And here is where we get back to diets. He says that as a general rule he's not a big fan of diet books. He says that most of the more successful ones are part of a larger marketing strategy to get people to buy stuff that is often little more than cheap junk food. He feels that a lot of this is part of the standard medical orthodoxy, and he isn't wild about it because it was this same orthodoxy that nearly killed him. He references the work of Gary Taubes (whose book we will also examine), who published the article "The Soft Science of Dietary Fat" in the journal *Science* as well as an article in the *New York Times Magazine* called "What If It's All Been a Big Fat Lie," and says this helped to shift attitudes on eating fat. He adds that despite all of this there are still many special-interest groups deeply invested in the high-carb, low-fat hypothesis. When I consider the vested interest of people like the processed food folks, agribusiness, and the Federal Government in much of this, I am pretty sure he's right.

Next we find another big reason for including this book. Remember that Bernstein is writing for people for whom information about diet can be crucial. If you really want to know what calories are and how they work you should read Chapter Three. I won't go into detail but basically what he is saying is that a calorie is a measure of energy when something is burned in a laboratory environment. A calorie, be it fat, protein or carbohydrate, doesn't act the same way in your body.

Next he looks at the Glycemic Index. He points out that this index was first conceived of by a Dr. David Jenkins (a person we have heard about before) around 1980. Jenkins was working on a way to test food that would be appropriate for diabetics. It would take two pages for me to try to describe the problems he feels exist with using the index (and I would probably only confuse the whole issue), but his final point is that he doesn't feel that it serves the needs of diabetics. He admits that he is in the minority in the diet field on this point, but if you are a diabetic, you should read all of his reasoning.

A last few odds and ends from this book that I didn't find elsewhere. For example, did you know that most of the sweeteners that claim to have zero calorie and zero carbs on their little packets contain some type of plain sugar as a bulk agent? So how can they can say zero carbs and zero calories? Because that federal watchdog the FDA says that if there are less than 0.9 grams, it doesn't have to be listed. Also, if you go on any of the low-carb diets, I would suggest getting his book for the list of what to eat and what not to eat because his lists are complete and specific. He says that he hasn't eaten fruit in 30 years. Cooked vegetables raise blood sugar faster than raw ones because the cooking coverts some of the cellulose to glucose (I didn't know until I read this why cooked carrots were sweeter than raw ones) and also makes them able to be digested more rapidly. He also has list of places to get all kinds of non-carb products.

One final comment. His coverage of the "thrifty genotype" is worth reading for all of those people who have real problems with weight. He says that an anthropologist named James V. Neel first used the term to help explain the extremely high incidence of Type Two diabetes and obesity in the Pima Indians in the southwestern United States. This is a condition that will be studied more and more as it might help to explain some ongoing weight problems.

EAT FAT, LOSE FAT

Dr. Mary Enig and Sally Fallon

To show a very different take on diet, our next book, *Eat Fat, Lose Fat*, is a bit farther out on the "edge" of the diet world. The authors start off by pointing out that "For the last 25 years, government recommendation, medical doctrine, food advertising, and so-called health experts have stressed low-fat and non-fat foods, cautioning people to avoid fats in general, particularly saturated fats from animal products and tropical fats, like coconut." Note the coconut reference because we will hear a lot more about that.

From the start they make a strong pitch for coconut oil and coconut foods. They say the secret to weight loss is feeling "satisfied" after eating. Their claim is that after eating coconut oil or other fats like those in butter, cream, nuts, meat and eggs, your body produces a hormone that tells you you're full. Like other diet books they slam trans fats but obviously don't follow the standard mantra on saturated fats.

When they get to their own diet suggestions, they give three possible approaches: The first they call "Quick and Easy Weight Loss." This is the only one that calls for calorie reduction. The next is named "Health Recovery," which is for people with special needs. And the last one, "Everyday Gourmet," they call their hearty maintenance program for life. All three of these include coconut oil (of course), cod-liver oil, and other fatty foods including butter, cream, whole milk, eggs, and meat. And about there they give a "case history" type of report, common to many diet books, that makes me want to raise an eyebrow. They tell us that one woman eliminated cellulite with their type of eating plan. I think that if they could prove that claim, there wouldn't be a coconut tree in the world safe from clamoring middle-aged women.

In Chapter Two called "Fats, the Real Deal," they say that it wasn't saturated fats that all of the "diet police" (their term) are so against that caused all of the obesity and health-related problems we see around us. They say the real bad guys are refined grains and sugars. They go to great lengths to examine the history of how we went from saturated fat to other types of food.

All of Chapter Three is about fat. In it they quote study after study that show that the intake of saturated fat does not correlate with heart attack deaths. They imply that this information has been "suppressed" and not given an honest hearing. They make some good points about whether or not cholesterol is the real culprit in heart disease. They back up these claims by citing studies that have been published in some of the top journals. One that caught my attention was the often quoted Framingham study. They say that this study did not show what was claimed by both the American Heart Association and the National Heart, Lung and Blood Institute in the articles these organizations published in the journal *Circulation*. In fact Enig and Fallon claim that the results show almost exactly the opposite! I don't know how valid their conclusions are, but I wish some well-qualified third party would look at their statements and confirm or deny them. As these two authors tell it, the claims they make seem to be well documented, if a bit off the wall. Although this book is not that well known, if you can find it, this chapter is well worth reading.

After reading page after page of study after study contradicting the standard approach to fats, cholesterol, and special diets they ask the logical question, why is this belief still in vogue? Their answer is that too many industries — drug, agribusiness, food processor, etc. — have profited mightily from this approach. An interesting aside on this is the pressure put on Dr. Enig in 1979 to stop her from publishing her findings regarding the problems with trans fats. They spend several pages telling the whole story of how she and others were pressured not to continue their work on the subject. Dr. Enig continued her research and worked for years to have trans-fat content listed on food labels.

Then the authors take the same tack often seen in diet books — criticize other diet authors. They cover Atkins (whose diet is something like theirs, but of course not as good) as well as Ornish with his low-fat vegetarian approach and the Sears' Zone diet. They also see problems with the South Beach Diet and Weight Watchers.

From there they move on to the specifics of their plan or "Phases," as they call them, all of which include coconut oil. This includes their "Special Weight-loss Tip" which is to drink one or two tablespoons of coconut oil twenty minutes before each meal. Then you will approach the meal with a diminished appetite. (This is not the first place that this has been recommended. In a book written some 50 years ago called *Calories Don't Count* by Herman Taller, M.D., he made the same recommendation.)

An interesting note they add on page 114 is why they don't think you should drink soy milk or eat soy products. They base this on the research done at the National Center for Toxicological Research that found that soy had a negative effect on the body's synthesis of a thyroid hormone. These researchers even went so far as to write to the FDA suggesting a health warning on these products. It didn't happen. Again, this is the only place I've run across a description of problems with soy. Considering the popularity of soy products it has to make you wonder.

From here on, it's about the standard approach, giving meal plans and recipes with suggestions as to where you can get some of the more esoteric products recommended. On the last two-and-a-half pages, they tell you how to use coconut oil for bath oil, wrinkles, acne, hair care, psoriasis, eczema, fungal infections, arthritis, warts, and even as a deodorant and insect repellent. (Wow!)

The big reason I included this book is because it is a very good example of authors, even those with good reputations such as these two, whipping one approach or product almost to death. This makes many people shy away from their ideas, many of which could well use more examination. Whether it is the fruit-juice diet, the cabbage-soup diet, or something else, when they say everyone else missed the boat and only they know the real elixir that will make you thin, rich, popular, or whatever, it raises questions. I'm not putting this book in the charlatan group because of the impressive reputations of the authors, and you can tell as you read that they have done their homework and have something important to say. However, when they, and others, start to pitch one particular food or product as the cure for almost everything you can't help but start to draw back. But I'll admit I didn't try their approach so I can't knock it from experience.

YOUNGER NEXT YEAR

Chris Crowley and Henry S. Lodge, M.D.

By now you might be getting a bit bored with the standard diet books. So for a change of pace let's look at a book that is much more of a "good health" book or more specifically a "get off your butt and stop just getting old" book. It is also the first book that I'm going to cover that as I read it, I kept thinking that I should recommend that you should read this book. But I ended up a bit less enthusiastic, and at the end of this review I'll tell you why. But there is a lot of good — no, excellent — stuff here, so let's cover that first. The central theme of this book, crudely put, is "To Hell with growing old gracefully." It is a lifelong plan to get up, get out, and get it on!

The two authors, an average guy and a respected doctor, more or less take turns writing chapter by chapter. Chris Crowley, the average guy, gets a bit too macho at times for my taste, but the doctor, Henry S. Lodge, provides some of the best advice on the "whys and hows" of good health I've run across. This statement of his is an eye-catcher: "What I am sure of is that there is a fundamental revolution at hand in the way people age."

Dr. Lodge starts off his chapter by saying that he has done a good job of what doctors do well in this country, which is treat people with disease. He goes on to say that in a way this is the wrong job. The right job? Keeping his patients healthy. He then makes the first of what will be many attention getting statements to be found in this book: "70 percent of premature death and aging is lifestyle-related." It gets even better when he adds: "we could eliminate more than half of all disease in men and women over 50. Not delay it, eliminate it." That's no small claim, but for the rest of the book he does an excellent job of showing how and why. The way to do this is not an easy task because, as the good doctor says, "As it turns out, health is biologically more complicated than disease." You can communicate with your body to obtain good health but it's not the standard "let's sit down and talk" type of communication. And he adds that left to its own devices, your body will simply fail to get the correct signals from today's world. But we can do a much better job of communicating with our bodies if we just take the time and make the effort.

I like this statement: "There's a critical distinction between aging and decay." He says aging is inescapable — decaying is not. So how does he advise us to learn the body code of communication and stop decay? He says the basic keys are daily exercise, emotional commitment, reasonable nutrition, and a real engagement with living. Then he adds, "But it starts with exercise." And he says it starts there because this signals the body to build. He goes on to give some examples of how and why this works, and has worked, for hundreds of thousands of years. He even explains how even during the bad times of winter, this basic brain uses even depression as a survival tool.

As he describes brain chemistry, he makes an obvious, but seldom heard, statement. The brain, not the rational everyday thinking part, but the part that controls all of the body processes, is deaf, dumb, and blind. (An interesting aside that he mentions: The only direct contact this part of the brain has to the outside world is the sense of smell.) And this "body brain" gets its basic signals from what you do. That body brain is perfectly adapted to the world that it grew up in over those hundreds of thousands of years. And without question, it believes what you "tell" it. The problem, the really big problem, is that the messages we send it from today's world are the wrong ones: Very little exercise, continuous stress, and, of course, a bad diet.

He then goes on to describe what he calls, "The Language of Nature." Snails and jellyfish developed most of the same stuff we did. Chemicals similar to Valium, adrenaline, cocaine and morphine are all natural products. No, that doesn't mean that the dope that the corner drug dealers are pushing is really health food. (Organic heroin – now there's a concept.) But the reason that street drugs have the effect they do is that we already have the receptacle sites built in and they are designed to respond to trace amount of these chemicals. The street variety slams them so hard they cause real damage. But the ones that your body can produce are of the right chemical content and amount. You get the right effects if (and that is one big "if") you send your body the right messages. And, again, it is the "body brain" that does all of this. On pages 44 and 45, he gives a full, factual description of this part of the brain and how it plays its role in our survival. In that long-ago world where it grew up, its single job was to keep you alive and reproducing. He says that after millions of years, when all of this worked so very well, we are the first creature to simply walk out of nature. And with that departure we produce the great health problems of our time: surfeit and idleness.

I would point out that, in a way, this could be expected. It was not against how that body brain was trained to survive. Because to accumulate that most precious of commodities, energy in the form of fat, that brain wanted us to eat as much as we could whenever we could, and rest whenever possible. So the basic problem was simple: We just got too successful at getting food with little effort. And since the basic problem is this "sit around and overeat" life style, what do we need to do? And here he is very specific: Exercise six days a week for the rest of your life! No, I wasn't that wild about that prescription either, but try as I might (and as lazy as I am,

107

believe me, I've looked), I couldn't find what I thought was a better answer.

In the next chapter Crowley gives a good rationale as to how to look at exercise. From childhood on there were things you "had" to do. When you were young, it was get up and go to school. Later it was, want to or not, get it out the door and to work. Well, exercise may well be as important, or even more important in the long run, than that. You simply have to see it like that. And it's here that I found a bit of advice that I would question. It comes from Crowley, and it is, "We urge you not to start gradually." I am sure that they are not advising a middle-aged person who is seriously overweight and out of shape to get out and put in a hard hour of exercise. In fact, on page 93, the authors point this out by saying, "Start out long and slow." I wish they had done a better job of explaining what seems to be conflicting advice. I believe what they meant was to commit to the six-day-a-week program. The statement that I do like is this one: "You're lucky that only one hour a day works so well."

Another "must do" statement from Crowley that I'm not so sure about is his declaration that you must join a gym. He goes into some length as to why he feels this is mandatory, and he does make some good points. But there are problems with this that he doesn't cover and when we get to my section of the book I'll go into this more in depth. When he talks about his own experience with spinning on page 87, it comes across as just plain macho stupid.

We now get to what I think is the best chapter in the book. It's written by Dr. Lodge and called "The Biology of Growth and Decay: Things That Go Bump in the Night." I won't go in depth here because you need to get this book and read this yourself. I don't care if you even were a biology major — I can almost guarantee you will gain a lot of information you didn't have before. For example, have you ever thought about heart attacks like this?: Heart attacks happen not because there is a problem with that wonderful muscle that beats around four billion times during your lifetime. The problem is circulation.

Another great source of information is Chapter Seven, "The Biology of Exercise." For example, the doctor gives an excellent description of why one type of exercise, where you really push it, burns glucose and why another type, low-intensity, light-aerobic exercise, burns fat. Lodge goes on to tell how and why this works this way. His message on diet is "Do not go on a diet, but quit eating crap" He says it is very simple: The message from thousands of studies, over decades of medical research, is clear: Never go on a diet again. Of course he is referring to the hundreds of "weight loss" diet plans that crowd the bookstore shelves. The alternative, as they have stressed throughout their book, is exercise and sensible eating. Be sure to read Chapter Fifteen, "The Biology of Nutrition: Thinner Next Year." I got a kick out of his comment on page 217 regarding not eating refined carbohydrates. He says, "How refreshing to have a major food fad turn out to be correct."

Now, since it has so much excellent information, and so many good ideas, what is my problem.

My big problem is really not with this book but with their next one that they did with the same title but added "*For Women.*" I have no objections to that approach. In fact it's a good marketing move. So, again, what's my problem? It's this: Why would you get someone like Gail Sheehy to write an introduction? This woman is one of the queens of the nifty mantras, New Wave auras, "get in touch with your feelings," and shakras all in a row, people. Remember me complaining about this approach from Dr Weil? Well, she is like a Dr Weil in overdrive without the brains or medical degree. In the introduction she talks about the "seasoned woman," who knows how to resonate with her sexuality. From her writings I can't help but feel that she is a "seasoned woman," who was left way too long in the marinade. She tells us that she had to have a "cranial sacral treatment," during which a "practitioner" listened with her hands and discovered that she had problems with the "energy and rhythmic patterns" in her body fluids. It seems that her last book had given her a "vicarious trauma." After finding out from this "practitioner" that the "important fluids" that were supposed to circulate between her head and her tail were moving sluggishly, she is off to learn "strip dancing" to release her inner goddess. And it goes on like that. It is my strongly held personal opinion that the 18-year-old can be very sexy and the intelligent 50-year-old can be very sexual. Maturing from one into the other is the true mark of the real adult in both men and women. So this life long "young sweetie" or "macho man" approach leaves me cold. But, like I said before, I'm old.

Just how much faith can you have in a physician who would permit this at the first of his book? I could see it from Crowley. From the way he writes, you get the feeling that all Sheehy had to do was stroke that over-active ego and he would have agreed. But not the doctor. From his writing I just can't help but feel he wasn't part of this deal.

Let me end this diatribe by saying I am probably so annoyed about this because their first book was so good. Still, I would encourage you to read their first book. It has just too much good stuff to pass up.

THE COMPLETE IDIOT'S GUIDE TO GLYCEMIC INDEX WEIGHT LOSS

Lucy Beale and Joan Clark

Next let's take a look at the new wave of diet books that are starting to use the Glycemic Index as the centerpiece of their diet plan. This book is from the *Complete Idiot's Guide* series and is called (no surprise here) *The Complete Idiot's Guide to Glycemic Index Weight Loss*.

The authors start by giving a brief history of how the Glycemic Index was developed. They say that the person who did some of the early work was Professor Thomas M.S. Wolever in the department of Nutritional Sciences at the University of Toronto. His work was mainly with people with Type Two diabetes. This was during the 1980s when almost every authority in the field of diet was prescribing a low-fat, high-carb diet. Finding problems with this diet for diabetics, he started to study which carbs increased blood sugar and insulin levels and which ones did not. From this he built the model for evaluating the foods that affected these values and determining how great the effect was. Next, Professor Jennie Brand-Miller from the University of Sydney picked up on this and did a much more complete list. There are some minor problems in the way the list is constructed, but it still remains one of the best guides available.

I'm not sure that Beale and Clark are on real solid ground when they say things like "most fruits, some whole grain products such as steel-cut oats and whole barley, and al dente pasta are low-glycemic foods." They even include legumes, dark chocolate, nuts, and seeds. And right here you run across what is often a problem with many of the Glycemic

Indexes. The reason that you can find quite a few differences between plans is simply because it is still fairly new. It takes time and money to do the laboratory work that is necessary to get a reading on any one food. Add to this the fact that any food can change its chemical content depending on where it was raised, how it was raised, and the overall conditions of harvesting and so on. Simply put, we are back to the same old "tomato A is often not the same as tomato B" problem. To give another example, sardines are usually listed as a type of fish high in oil. But caught at different times they can have as little as only two percent oil content. Like almost everything else about food, there is very little that is always 100 percent true.

Next they get to "Glycemic Load," which is the logical next step. This is simply a way of saying not just what kind but also how much. They get the glycemic load by taking the Glycemic Index of a food, multiplying it by the quantity in grams and dividing by 100. This may sound a bit confusing, but it would seem that the best advice is that the amount of anything that you eat has its limits.

Then they do something that I like very much. They say that all of this is still in development and has some unanswered questions like: How much does fat lower the index? Why does cinnamon lower the index? And a number of other "whys." They also include their own food pyramid which is not even close to the new one from the U.S.

government. They advise you not to be in a big hurry to lose weight because if you take it off slowly there is a better chance that it will stay off. This is so much better than the "lose ten pounds in ten minutes" kind of pitch you so often hear from the weight-loss crowd.

In Chapter Nine they pretty much show that this is a "weight loss for women" kind of book. The title of the chapter "Get Your Mind Aligned" gets pretty close to the Dr. Phil approach. They want you to "Harness your mental powers, write weight-loss affirmations, banish past weight loss failures, and connect with new ways of eating." I'm not saying that it's wrong, I'm just saying that to me it sounds like it is approaching the all-too-standard psycho-babble .

Another problem is that, when it comes to what and how much to eat, they want "about three or four ounces of animal protein and two or three servings of vegetables." And then they suggest you look at how much space things take up on your plate and allocate accordingly. They say that you can forget about that 16-ounce steak unless you plan to feed four or five people. A lot of this has a "Zone diet" sound to it.

When it comes to describing the different kinds of fats, theirs is about the best I've seen. If you are a bit confused about omega-3s and 6s and all the rest, here is a good place to find the answers. And this is also true as they go on to other foods. For example, their take on soy. Many diet plans are wild for soy products of all kinds. They take a much closer look. They don't say it's bad, but they do point out things that could be a problem for some people.

Then it's on to things like sugar and junk food. If you get a chance, read pages 136 and 137 on how to tell if it's junk food. This is both clever and excellent. For example, they say that if your children beg you to buy it, it's probably junk. They then add, "We have never yet met a child who begged for string beans." Also, this book not only has a good index, but also has an appendix which lists the Glycemic Index and the glycemic load for a large number of carbohydrates. This listing alone is worth the price of the book.

EAT, DRINK, AND BE HEALTHY

Walter C. Willett, M.D.

This is the most informative book of all that we have covered. The author is involved with many of the big studies like the Framingham study and the Harvard Nurses' Study. He has a tremendous amount of information available to him and knows how to express it in a readable form. He was trained in one of our country's best medical schools, has practiced both here and in Third World countries, and is considered by many to be the best authority in the field of nutrition. I will disagree with him on some points and do my best to explain why. But it would be wise to remember that he is the expert and I am not. All things considered, this is an excellent book.

In the preface he describes how one of his reasons for writing this updated version of his previous book was to "challenge the misleading advice embodied in the U.S. Department of Agriculture's ubiquitous Food Guide Pyramid." (Note: this book was published before the USDA changed their diet suggestions once again but kept with the same overall philosophy.) He points out that "Politics and business, as usual, ultimately trumps science," and he feels that the new "My Pyramid" offers even less guidance than the one before it. He says that he will try to do what he can to show how and where they were wrong. As he notes in Chapter One, the new "My Pyramid" did more to help agribusiness and food companies than it did to help you. He warns to keep in mind that this document was developed by the same agency in the Federal Government that is responsible for promoting American agriculture and that your good health is not their first priority. Sadly, this is not the first time we have heard this.

You should consider reading this book for a number of reasons, but the big one, to me, is the background that he gives on just how things like "My Pyramid" are developed by the government. For example, in 2003, when they needed to hire a new executive director for the center, they picked a man who was an expert in animal, not human, nutrition. Whose job experience included employment at the National Livestock and Meat Board, the National Pork Producers Association, and the National Pork Board. Willett doesn't just give some vague reasons for what happened as "My Pyramid" was being put together but shows specifically where they made mistakes and why this is not of casual importance. The new "Pyramid" is not just for those who might want to use it. The big problem is that it now sets the standard for all federal as well as state nutritional programs. For what? For things like food stamps, school lunch programs, the armed forces, and others.

Willett starts with a list of problems with the old USDA program: First, it says that all fats are bad. The truth is that not all are bad. In fact some are not only good for you but important for good health. Second, all carbohydrates are good for you. The truth is that some are good, some not so good, and some bad. Third, protein sources are interchangeable. He says no. Fourth, dairy products are essential. He says it's calcium that you need and there are as good or better sources. Fifth, eat your potatoes. He says only if you are physically active then it could be all right but not for the rest of us. And sixth, they didn't say anything about weight, exercise, alcohol, or vitamins. The new pyramid, he says, includes some advances over the old. Yes, they now say there are some good oils, but they still lump all proteins together. And they still recommend three servings of milk or other dairy products a day. He sees a big problem with the vertical stripe plan and thinks it's more confusing than helpful.

Then we get to his own plan, which he calls "The Healthy Eating Pyramid." And he tells you up front that his plan is not set in stone. He says the reason it's not is because there is still lots to be learned about nutrition. But he does feel that it is the best plan around, and he spends most of the book showing you why. Here are the big things as he sees them: 1.Watch your weight. 2. Eat fewer bad fats and more good ones. 3. Eat more whole-grain products and fewer refined ones. 4. Choose healthier sources of proteins. (He is not a red meat fan.) 5. Eat plenty of vegetables and fruits, but hold the potatoes. 6. Use alcohol in moderation. 7. Take a multivitamin for insurance. I think that for most people this is a plan that they can stick with.

In Chapter Two, "What Can You Believe About Diet?," he lists a number of contradictory statements that have been made about what to eat or not to eat. He quotes a good line from an Ellen Goodman article where she writes, "There seems to be some sort of planned obsolescence now to medical news. Today's cure is tomorrow's poison pellet. Fresh research has a sell-by date that is shorter than the one on the cereal box." He adds that the mountains of media of all kinds don't help. And here he gets to a point that is too seldom made:

"Fifty years ago medical research mostly ignored nutrition." He says this has gotten better and the interest of the general public has increased. But that means that media of all kinds jump on the smallest steps in research and trumpet them as major advances and breakthroughs when in fact they may just be only tentative findings. And so when it comes to reporting health information, if it sounds good, and even better, contradictory, why then get it out there. The vast majority of people in the news field have very little scientific background. This means that they judge more on what is attention-getting than what is fact. And this makes trying to get valid health news out to the public just that much more difficult.

In the first chapter, we hit a piece of information that should be done in needlepoint and put on every person's wall if that individual is in any way involved with giving information or advice regarding nutrition. This statement is part of a section called "working with real people poses special challenges." He makes several great points, including the following: "The foods you eat each day contain thousands of different natural chemicals, some known and well studied, some known and unstudied, many completely unknown and unmeasurable." And there you have the honest truth about the study of nutrition. And why the hundreds of diet, health or nutrition books that are out there need to be looked at with a very critical eye. He goes on to tell how different studies are done and why all of them have their own problems. If you want to get a rough idea of how many studies and how big they are, the problems they have, and how long they take, then look at page 32 where he lists some of these.

Chapter Three starts with weight. He says try not to gain weight and lose a few if you're too heavy. He points out that this is not a new, exciting idea that is going to get him on *The Oprah Winfrey Show* but it is at the center of how to prevent a lot of health problems in the future. He gives several ways to evaluate your weight, but one that is an eye-catcher is to compare your weight now to what it was at the age of 21. He says it has probably changed but you would be a lot healthier if it hadn't. Next he examines where you store your fat: Is it around your waist and chest or your hips and thighs? If it is around your waist and chest it may be more of a health problem. He isn't a big fan of the "hip to waist" approach that you hear a lot about these days. He does say, however, that it is worth looking into as it can be a helpful guide.

After this section he gets back on the "calorie-is-a-calorie" approach. It is here that he gets into the different kinds of popular diets, and shows their good and bad sides. He does say that low-fat diets are not the answer and that low-carb diets may help. No, he's not an Atkins fan, but he thinks that even Atkins was headed away from saturated fat before his untimely death. He does like the Glycemic Index idea. As he points out, people with diabetes have been using it for years, and he notes how the index is now moving into the mainstream diet field.

Then he gives you his "Three steps to weight control" which are: 1. If you are not physically active, then get moving. 2. Find an eating plan that works for you. 3. Become a defensive eater. He then goes to some length to explain each one. But first he says, "I wish I could give you a more precise set of instructions guaranteed to control weight. But I can't." People are just too different to expect one plan to work for all. But he can, and does, give you a number of good strategies that have worked for others.

When it comes to exercise, he says that it counts the most when it comes to good health. He gives a list, and it is a long one, of just what exercise can do and how it helps. One of several suggestions is walking. As you read today's health gurus you'll notice that walking has become the "go to" exercise for a lot of people in this field. The problem is that people don't walk, they stroll, and believe that they are getting the job done. Willett points out that when he says walking he means move! He says to walk like you were late to a meeting at about 100 steps a minute or a clip of three or four miles an hour. Try walking at this pace, and you will find it is much faster than normal walking. He says that intensity matters and it should be for a minimum of 30 minutes a day.

When it comes to a specific diet he says that one low in refined carbohydrates is the best bet. He likes something like the Mediterranean type diet with plenty of vegetables and moderate amounts of whole grains (note that he says "moderate amounts of whole grains") and relatively little red meat. Next is defensive eating. He says that, sure, you have to watch what kind of food you eat but it also means watching how much you eat. He says to be selective and choose small portions and beware of desserts. Slow down and pay attention to your food when you eat. He goes on with a lot of other good suggestions and why and how they can help. Then we get to the section, page 58-65, where he goes into the pluses and minuses of almost all of the diet plans you can name and some you have never heard of (and does a much better job than I am doing). His comment on Dr. Phil's diet plan: "The closest this plan comes to offering nutritional advice is promoting foods that take a long time to prepare and eat."

In Chapter Four, "Surprising News About Fat," he gives the following facts: People on low-fat diets generally lose about two to four pounds after several weeks, but then gain that weight back even while continuing with the diet. In country-to-country surveys across Europe, women with the lowest fat intake are the most likely to be obese, while those with the highest fat intake are the least likely to be fat.. He notes that in the United States, the gradual reduction in the fat content of the average diet, from 40 percent of calories to about 33 percent, has been accompanied by a gradual increase in the average weight and a dramatic increase in obesity. From there he goes on to give an excellent description of the different kinds of fats and why you need some kinds of fat in your diet and not others. He then gives a complete description of what each kind of fat does in the body. It's no surprise that trans fats are not his favorite. But his final verdict is that for good health we need some fat in our diet and most of it should not be saturated.

Then on to Chapter Five, "Carbohydrates for Better and Worse." This is pretty much what you would expect. However, he goes deeper into things like not just the Glycemic Index but also glycemic load. He is specific about the effect of high-carb diets on people who are already overweight, and it's pretty much all bad. It is in this chapter that he goes back to the Glycemic Index and takes it a step further with his description of the glycemic load. He does a good job of showing why both of these should be taken into consideration. Again, let me encourage you to read this book. There is just nothing else that I've seen that goes into this kind of depth regarding these subjects and explains them as well as he does.

And then we get to proteins. He starts this chapter by saying, "We know far less about protein in healthy diets and the role it plays in the onset of disease than we do about fats and carbohydrates." To give you an idea how difficult a study like this can be, consider the fact that there are at least ten thousand different proteins in the human body. And although the nutritionists have an idea what the minimum amount needed may be, there is not a conclusion as to the ideal amount for good health. Then Willett addresses the ongoing argument regarding the source of the protein that we eat and shows how it plays out on two levels: personal health and environmental health. He is pretty even in his presentation but in the end it is the plant protein that comes out on top from an environmental point of view. (There is a reason that he, like many other nutritionists, take this approach. I'll go deeper into the "why" in the last section of this book.) The big problem with animal protein is saturated fat. His final suggestion is to mix up your proteins and balance them with carbs.

Next it's on to his coverage of vegetables, fruit, nuts, juices, etc.. Again he gives you a good detailed look at what they may do (and he says "may") for overall good health. This is not the "broccoli will cure everything" approach. He simply tells you what is known and why these things should be in your diet. Also he tells you why giving advice or doing research on these foods is so difficult: None stay the same. It's back to the tomato problem again. I could go one for another two or three pages to tell you how he tells you how to put it all together, but it is best for you to, once again, read this book.

GOOD CALORIES, BAD CALORIES

Gary Taubes

This is the last book that we are going to examine. If you want a real grip on the "whys" when it comes to many of the strange things that are happening in the field of diet today, you will find them in this book. We will only look at some of the highlights.

Remember the story about the boy who pointed out that the Emperor had no clothes? Well, Taubes is the person who points out that many diet experts may well be intellectually naked. A complaint often heard about his work is that he "lacks the formal training for this enterprise." In response it's fair to note that the boy who outed the Emperor's lack of wardrobe didn't have a Ph.D. in clothing design.

Taubes is a science writer, a very good one, who has spent years looking behind the scenes of different areas of nutrition. He is the only writer to win the Science-in-Society award three times from the National Association of Science Writers, which is the maximum number of wins they allow. I think that when he decided to write this book he knew it was going to be controversial so he made it a point to "over-research" almost every statement. This means that the book gets a bit dry in spots, but perhaps he felt that he didn't have a choice.

He opens with a Prologue, and be sure to read this. It includes some of the best history available regarding diets. For example, he covers not only the Banting diet that we've seen before but others like *The Physiology of Taste* by Brillat-Savarin, published in 1825, that advises that to lose weight, don't eat bread, rice, potatoes or sugar. It also says to stay away from anything "starchy or floury." It sounds like today's low-carb crowd had a distant intellectual relative. Also in the Prologue he quotes Harvard nutritionist Jean Mayer, who says, "To attribute obesity to overeating is as meaningful as to account for alcoholism by ascribing it to over drinking." Taubes goes on to list a number of other professional people and world-wide organizations that, at the time, had positive things to say about a low-carbohydrate type of eating plan. But then in the 1970s things started to change.

In 1973, at the first conference hosted by the National Institutes of Health, Taubes says that the only talk on obesity was given by a Cornell University nutritionist, Charlotte Young, who had been treating obesity for 20 years. She referenced the work of Margaret Ohlson, head of the Department at Michigan State University, who had also tested carb-restricted diets in the 1950s and had gotten good results. But also in 1973 the American Medical Association published an editorial branding low-carb diets as "a dangerous fad." Which brings up the question — why this great change?

Taubes spends the rest of the book doing an excellent job of trying to answer this question. To quote him early in the book: "The reason for this book is straightforward: despite the depth and certainty of our faith that saturated fat is the nutritional bane of our lives and that obesity is caused by overeating and sedentary behavior, there has always been copious evidence to suggest that those assumptions are incorrect, and that evidence is continuing to mount."

But the low-fat diet, as the solution, did happen and became more and more entrenched. In the 1980s The Surgeon General's Report on Nutrition and Health recommended a low-fat diet. The USDA came out with its food pyramid, which also praised a low-fat, high- carbohydrate eating plan. And so the low-fat craze was underway.

It is also in the Prologue that he brings up what could be some of the most important information to be found in the book. And that is: Long before what he calls the "low-fat-is-good-health dogma," there had been another hypothesis, proposed by many people who had spent decades in the field. It concerned something we have heard before called the "diseases of civilization" (heart disease, diabetes, colorectal and breast cancer, tooth decay, etc.), which they felt were products of diet. You should hear a lot more about this in coming years, as it seems to produce a great many sensible suggestions. As mentioned before, Taubes does the heavy lifting when it comes to giving the background on present thinking about obesity and heart disease. He shows how most of today's beliefs are pretty much based on guesses and mythology. For example, he says that the Framingham report did not show what the published data often claimed that it did. (This isn't the first place we've run across that statement.) And that is only one of many slips in research that he uncovers.

On the first page of Chapter Three we find the statements that will set the stage for the "Diet Wars" over the next thirty-five years. These include things like Paul Ehrlich's book *The Population Bomb*, which warned about over-population; statements from people like Jean Mayer, from Harvard, pointing out that to feed the hungry of the world we needed to "simplify" our diet; and a surprising best seller by twenty-six year-old vegetarian Francis Moore Lappé called *Diet for a Small Planet*. Books like these, and others with a strong vegetarian slant, had a major impact on both academia and the general public. On page 44, Taubes gives January 14, 1977, the same date that we saw in Pollan's book, as the date which marked a major change in the approach to diet. This was the date that Senator George McGovern announced the publication of the first *Dietary Goals for the United States*. This document stressed the risk factors regarding the consumption of fat. This then became the standard approach, not just for government agencies, but for the popular press as well. Taubes notes that at the time that the above was published the National Academy of Science Director Donald Fredrickson said, "We shouldn't touch it with a ten-foot pole. We should let the crazies on the Hill say what they want." Taubes also give a quote from the president of the same group, Philip Handler, as calling it "nonsense."

From the start, problems cropped up with the stress on a low-fat diet when it didn't produce the results expected. For example data from the 1982 Harvard Nurses' Study didn't show that eating less fat produced less breast cancer. In fact, the women who ate more fat had slightly fewer tumors. Also, the Framingham Study published findings in 1987 that looked at another side of the diet debate, cholesterol, and showed that those results also ran counter to expectations. Its results showed that men under the age of 50 with high cholesterol were more prone to premature death. But, and here is the part that is seldom mentioned, over the age of 50, in both men and women, life expectancy showed no correlation with high or low cholesterol. Furthermore, people whose cholesterol declined during the study were more likely to die prematurely than those whose cholesterol increased or stayed the same.

Even as far back as 1966, the book *Diabetes, Coronary Thrombosis and the Saccharine Disease* by Campbell and Cleave showed that their research seemed to indicate that these problems stemmed from combining refined carbohydrates with saturated fat. At the same time most of the big names in the field were saying that fat alone was the problem. At first it was all fats. But in the last few years, as we have seen in some of the previous reviews, many have changed this to "some fats are necessary for good health." But not saturated fat.

Taubes makes it plain that this was not just a disagreement on something as simple as how to lose a few pounds before swimsuit season. This conflict of ideas, which still goes on today, was about how certain foods affect not just body weight but basic health. In fact, Thomas Cleave, the co-author of the above book, went so far as to call many health problems "refined-carbohydrate diseases." He got a lot of criticism for this belief, but answered by saying that he thought it was plainly naive to think otherwise. Cleave also noted that in regard to carbohydrates, the refining process did its damage in three ways. (It is interesting that he stressed this over 40 years ago.) First, he said that it caused over-eating because the body was fooled by the drastic change in the calories-per-volume of the processed food. Sugar being a good example. You would have to chew a big bunch of sugarcane or sugar beets to get the same amount that is in one tablespoon of the refined product. Second, this refining process removed nutrients and fiber that were in the original plant. And third, this processing increased the rate of digestion in an unnatural way compared to the consumption of the original plant. His biggest single belief, which has been ignored, was that mixing refined carbs with any kind of fat was the primary problem. For years most of the researchers in the diet field made no major distinction between carbohydrates that were refined and those that were not. Even as late as 1989, when the National Academy of Science published Diet and Health guide they lumped them together.

This refined versus unrefined controversy wasn't by any means new ground. As far back as the early 1950s John Yudkin, who founded the first Department of Nutrition at Queen Elizabeth College in London, had written a book called *This Slimming Business*. This, along with one called *Pure, White and Deadly*, which he wrote after retiring in 1972, lambasted refined carbohydrates, with a stress on the dangers of processed sugar. In fact, his constant stress that sugar alone was the primary problem and that saturated fat did not increase cholesterol made nutritionists start to disparage his research to the point that it became counter-productive to even reference his work.

Then came the fabulous 1960s, and along with sex, drugs, and rock and roll, came fiber. Taubes shows how the ideas flowing from this era did a nice job of dovetailing with the ideas of people like Burkitt and Trowell, who looked to fiber as the answer to health problems. This had a clever way of pushing Cleave's refined carbs ideas aside by saying that the problem with refined carbs was not that it was sugar or grain but that it was the loss of fiber from refining. This had a "back to nature" ring to it that did a nice job of fitting in with the attitude of the times. Taubes then devotes a whole chapter to fiber because it was the next "new, new thing" to hit the diet field and is still a big number today. Why the big shift? Because it fits neatly with two ideas. First, the "fat is bad" crowd was having trouble correlating their beliefs with the fact that cultures that ate fat, sometimes a lot of fat, didn't have the diseases that should go with that diet. They came up with a lot of reasons for this, none of which seemed to fit all that well. And then along came fiber, which they felt could answer a lot of the problems. Second, and from the impact on the public's point of view, the diet of the counterculture provided a nice fit. Veggies, legumes, and grains became the preferred diet of people in the counterculture crowd as well as of movie stars and many in academia who were in the diet field. Kind of a "bridge over organic grain fields," you might say.

Let me quote directly from his book. On page 124 Taubes writes, "The fiber hypothesis and the refined-carbohydrate hypothesis of chronic disease were photographic negatives of each other." He points out that the fiber idea hit big, despite the fact that the refined-carb idea was the only one supported by the evidence. One of the claims regarding the benefit of fiber was that it would reduce the incidence of colon cancer. But a $30 million trial done by the National Cancer Institute confirmed that fiber had no effect on colon cancer.

As early as page four the name Ancel Keys comes up. He was at the University of Minnesota in the 1960s and first came to public prominence when he appeared on the cover of *Time* magazine. In the accompanying article he stressed a low-fat, low-cholesterol diet. President Eisenhower had a heart attack that year so diet was much in the news. Keys, probably more than any other one person, made fat — at first all fats and now saturated fat as well as dietary cholesterol — the villains. No matter what research counters his claims, his ideas, in one form or another, still affect much of the thinking on diet today. And since Dr. Keys lived to be over 100 years old, one has to be a little hesitant to criticize his diet ideas.

Then in the chapter "Triglycerides and Cholesterol," Taubes gives some fascinating information regarding research that was done as far back as 1961 by some pretty big names in the field. People like the Nobel laureate Joseph Goldstein, Peter Kuo, and others did research built on work done by Margaret Albrink, who at the time was at Yale. This involved the study of cholesterol and triglycerides and their effect on heart disease. The gist of it was that triglycerides were a more important factor in heart disease than cholesterol. They also found that a low-carbohydrate diet was beneficial in lowering this risk factor. After their research was published by the American Medical Association, it asked if too many people had boarded the "cholesterol bandwagon."

But by then the Keys crowd had many more people from their camp doing mountains of research on the cholesterol/fat hypothesis and so they continued, as they still do today, to dominate the academic field. Also, and this perhaps should receive more stress than it has, back then cholesterol was easy to measure in blood samples. But there were few places that had the equipment to do the complex testing then needed to measure triglycerides. For this reason, the mass data studies that were being done included only cholesterol.

Let's skip over to the next chapter "The Role of Insulin." By now Taubes has taken us into a discussion of both the metabolic syndrome (problems caused by diet) and small, dense LDL particles. If you have cholesterol problems, this is the chapter where you will find information that I doubt you have seen before. And as you read this you have to wonder why this isn't better known.

When he gets to the chapter called "Sugar," he hits what you feel must be his own personal complaint. He is allergic to high-fructose corn syrup, but that doesn't mean that he is alone in his objections to this product. Regular table sugar and HFCS have been the subject of more and more research, and the results have been consistently negative regarding their impact on health. Because of the confusion in the minds of many on the effects of fructose, sucrose, and glucose on the body, most of us lump them all together. Taubes shows how this happens and why this misconception may be dangerous. He concludes that high-fructose corn syrup may be more of a problem than we are aware. An interesting point regarding this potential problem: There is some research which shows a rather impressive correlation between the consumption of sugar and cancer. It is worth noting here that the industry that produces high-fructose corn syrup has, at this writing, started an advertising campaign in which they stress that it is nothing more than a sweetener from a healthy product, corn. It is highly probable that this expenditure of millions of advertising dollars will pay off for this industry.

In Chapter Fourteen, "The Mythology of Obesity," he points out, as have those before him, that the closer you look at the problem of obesity the more complex it becomes. He quotes a National Academy of Science report that says, "Most studies comparing normal and overweight people suggest that those who are overweight eat fewer calories than those of normal weight." But it is still the common belief in the field of nutrition that, without question, obesity is caused by overeating as expressed in the calories-in-and-calories-out theory.

The general approach to the whole question of overweight and obesity has a rather bizarre history. If you think that the cabbage soup diet was a bit odd, how about an approach used in the early 1800s, such as causing bleeding from the jugular and/or applying leeches to the anus, which was supposed to aid in weight loss. Also the drinking of vinegar was a popular diet craze until it started killing people. These diet plans may be only slightly more unsound than some of the suggestions that you can find in diet books today. This leads to Chapter Fifteen, "Hunger," where we get to many of the basic problems surrounding diets of all kinds if the purpose is to lose weight. Again and again, researchers who tried to establish realistic weight-loss programs kept running into a number of problems. The point made is quite simple: There is much more going on here than simply "calories in and out."

This doesn't mean that people in the diet field have given up on the low calorie intake approach. Taubes mentions the *Handbook of Obesity*, published in 1998 and edited by George Bray, Claude Bouchard and W.P.T. James, in which the authors note that calorie-restricted diets are the cornerstone of weight reduction. But later in the book they admit that diets of this type "are known to be poor and not long-lasting." Taubes also quotes an experiment done at the Mayo Clinic in which sixteen healthy people were overfed a thousand calories a day, in addition to their regular diet. Their weight gain varied from one pound to almost nine pounds. This puts some question marks to the hard-and-fast rule of the simple calories-in-and-out approach. Next we hear about Louis Newburgh, a professor of medicine at the University of Michigan, and his hard-line belief that obesity was caused by nothing more than gluttony and sloth. He was pushing this point of view as far back as the 1930s, with anecdotal evidence which he said proved his point. And so the concept of the "perverted appetite" is still sometimes quoted as a cause of overweight.

It is pretty obvious that the standard diet book that promotes any kind of calorie restricted diet — and most do in one guise or another — simply does not tell the whole story. But, if you go to the average doctor for advice or take a course in nutrition at most colleges or universities, this is the advice you will get. Taubes does not go as deeply as he could have in addressing this problem. For the person involved with diet and/or weight loss, this answer is important. Because the nutrition crowed has failed on this issue, they more or less just hunkered down and even in the face of this failure, kept chanting their calories-in-and-out nutritional rosary. But because the need still exists for answers that work, people in the field of psychology and psychiatry have tried to pick up the slack. This produced not only the unfortunate books like the "Dr. Phil" fiasco but some very good ones like Deirdre Barrett's *Waistland*.

As you can tell I was very impressed with Taubes' book, and it would be easy to go on for many more pages discussing it. But I'm afraid that, once again, the best answer is for you to read this yourself. I would add one last comment: Take a close look at page 293 where he shows the problems of trying to use thermodynamics, as is often done by the calories-in-and-out group, to explain how the body uses food and why it doesn't work.

A QUICK LOOK AT SOME OTHER DIET BOOKS

If you look at the diet books section of any large bookstore you will see shelf after shelf of new "breakthrough" books on health and diet. For example, Oz and Roizen have been quite successful with their series of books that start with "You" in the title. In fact, it looks like they have joined Atkins, Sears, Agatston, and a few others that have gone from being authors to being an industry. Dr. Oz has authored or co-authored several books and a column for a men's magazine and has become a regular on television. He does a good job of explaining how our bodies work but really doesn't have that much new to add to diet knowledge. But he does stress exercise and explains the Glycemic Index during his television show. Also he is sincere in his beliefs, looks good on television, has Oprah's endorsement and gives a lot of attention to the "spiritual side" of good health, which is becoming popular again after having been a staple of the 1960s.

A newer diet book that also brings "spiritual" into dieting is *Quantum Wellness: A Practical and Spiritual Guide to Health and Happiness* by Kathy Freston, with a forward by Dr. Oz. She also wrote *The One: Discovering the Secrets of Soul Mate Love* as well as *A Miracle: Seven Spiritual Steps to Finding the Right Relationship*. Another book, *Eat This, Not That!* by David Zinczenko, with Matt Goulding, is one of the few diet books aimed specifically at men. Another is the *GenoType Diet* by Dr. Peter J. D'Adamo, with Catherine Whitney. The good doctor D'Adamo is a naturopathic physician who, like several others in the field, has jumped on the human genome idea and used it to construct diet plans for different "types" of people. Then there is *The Ultimate Tea Diet* by Mark Ukra, or as he calls himself, Dr Tea. He champions a well-balanced diet combined, no surprise here, with lots of tea. *Slim for Life*, by Dr. Gillian McKeith, is a compendium of much of what you have seen before but done in an appealing way. She says you should exercise every day.

The above is only a very short list of what is available now, with more being added each day. From the first diet book to require calorie counting written in 1918 by Lulu Peters, up to the *No-Fad Diet* put out by the American Heart Association, which has the same calorie counting requirements, this approach still remains popular. It is interesting that the American Heart Association book not only sticks to the timeworn calorie-counting approach but has only 79 pages of text in a 445- page book. The rest of the book, like those written by many of their peers, is filled with recipes, lists, and charts.

The big change that has happened over the last twenty years is what might be called the Atkins or Agatston approach with Agatston's The South Beach Diet plan probably having the biggest effect because of the exclusion of saturated fat. You can see this change in books like *The Wall Street Diet* by Heather Bauer, who calls things like white bread, white pasta, bagels, muffins, etc. "dry carbs" and says that they should be avoided if the object is to lose weight.

Another approach that is gaining in popularity shows up in books like *The Volumetrics Weight-Control Plan: Feel Full on Fewer Calories* by Dr. Barbara J. Rolls, a professor of behavioral health at Penn State. You might call this "calorie counting mixed with semi-vegetarian eating." She started a recent speech by saying that the laws of thermodynamics have not been reversed so calories are the answer. The plan is basically fruits, vegetables and soups so that you fill up on foods large in volume but low in calories.

Considering Dr. Rolls' approach to calories, perhaps we should again mention a book written almost 50 years ago called *Calories Don't Count* by Herman Taller, M.D., which addressed the role of carbohydrates in weight gain a number of years before it became popular. His premise was that consumption of fats could cause weight loss and that this, and not calorie counting, was the secret to weight control.

Building Your Own Collection

Often, as a book is being examined, my comments have included something like "You should read this." If you are really serious about a wise eating plan, then it calls for more attention to the works of others than I have even begun to cover here. I strongly recommend that you get books like *Younger Next Year* as well as those that we looked at by Willett and Taubes. I only scratched the surface of these excellent books so reading them yourself is highly recommended. Also in your own collection should be the 16th edition of a book called Barbara Kraus' *Calories and Carbohydrates*. First published in 1973 this is the best collection of information on both calories and carbs that I have found.

Should you decide that a vegetarian or Mediterranean diet is more to your liking then the latest books by Mollie Katzen, one of the best selling cookbook authors, should be on your list. Best known for her *The Moosewood Cookbook*, a vegetarian cookbook first published in 1977, she has also written several others. The one I would recommend is her latest, which includes comments by Dr. Willett. With the addition of Dr. Willett, there are also some fish and chicken cooking suggestions.

Finally let me add a personal plea: Don't make the centerpiece of your diet and exercise plan nothing more than an obsession with personal appearance! A pop star body or six-pack abs may be the emphasis of many of the quick weight loss diets, but the vast majority of us just are not built that way in the first place. You hear little about it, but there truly are different types of body builds. The terms endomorph and ectomorph seem to have fallen out of our vocabulary when discussing body types. But it is a simple fact that high-chested, slender-waisted movie star idols are far from the average body type. If you hold your weight down and eat and exercise wisely you will look good, but more importantly, you will be healthy.

SOME POSSIBLE CONCLUSIONS

Moving On

We have discussed enough diet plans of the last 50 years or more to show the lack of agreement about what is best. Jeffrey Friedman, an obesity researcher at Rockefeller University, points out that "everyone has a deeply held set of beliefs about the cause of obesity but there is little objective scientific support for any of them." This would seem to the casual observer to be a rather strange situation. Why can't the researchers involved just do their jobs and come to a unanimous decision about the best kind of diet? The answer is this: To get these kinds of absolute answers it would require taking 20,000 randomly selected babies at birth and keeping them in a controlled environment for the next 90 to 100 years You could then end up with some hard data. Since this isn't going to happen, the best that can be done is something like the Framingham or Harvard Nurses' Study. This provides a lot of "soft" data. The data is soft because it depends on the honesty and memory of a large number of people. And it is sad but true, that the three things that people lie about the most are money, sex, and diet. So you end up with the kinds of disagreements that we have just examined.

In an attempt to do something close to the huge research study suggested above, the National Children's Study, which is connected to the National Institute of Child

Health and Human Development, plans to follow 100,000 children from before birth to the age of 21 to try to get some kind of handle on what really happens. This would seem to be a step in the right direction.

But let's move on and try to put together what we do know and see if we can't come up with some practical suggestions on a diet for the individual.

First a Bit of Background

Perhaps the best place to start is to describe you, the human being, from both a biological and historical perspective. We will take a look far back into your own genetic history because it will have a lot to do with diet. Have you happened to notice that you, along with other humans, don't have fur? Also, you have a bigger collection of sweat glands than any other primate. That odd bare-body quality is one of the traits that helped get you here. In fact, you probably wouldn't be here if it weren't for that semi-hairless body. The following is not some break-through idea of my own. Others with better credentials than mine, such as Deirdre Barrett, Ph.D. in her book *Waistland,* have come to much the same conclusion.

Let's also look at another fact about your anatomy. Compare your body to all the other primates and you're the one with the big butt. No, I'm not talking about what you have managed to add over the last 20 or 30 years. I'm referring to those excellent gluteus maximus muscles. And there's more. Those thigh muscles are also top of the line. Oh, and let's not forget the calf muscles and those best-of-class Achilles tendons as well as the tendons in the foot, all designed for running. Even the inner ear is an aid to balance while on the move. This is not an original idea on my part either. Biology professor Dennis Bramble from the University of Utah and anthropologist Dan Lieberman from Harvard published an interesting article called "How Running Made Us Human" in the magazine *Discover* covering this in much greater detail.

Now put all of those things together along with several other refinements and what you have is a well-designed body that a ruthless killer can use to run down almost any other land animal on earth over distance and time. That's right. You, the champion of the recliner and remote control, were designed to be the victor, many thousands of years ago, in a race where the loser died and the winner got dinner.

And it's still true today. There used to be a 100-mile race in California that stretched from the high mountains to the low desert, which included both people and horses. The horses never even came close to winning. For another example, go down to the Copper Canyon country of northern Mexico and check out the games that the Tarahumara Indians play. The men run and kick a ball over an 80- to 100-mile course. The women, being a much gentler sex, only run a 40-mile course clad in homemade sandals while rolling a hoop.

I can add a bit of family history to the feats of the Tarahumara. Back in the early 1900s, both my father and father-in-law managed mines in northern Mexico. Like other mine managers around them, they hired these people as messengers because the mines would usually be many miles from the nearest town where they could get mail and order supplies. They would send the runners to pick up mail and to place orders with the merchants, who would then deliver by mule. I have heard my father say that there wasn't a horse alive that could beat these runners over a distance of 50 miles or more of fairly smooth going. And, when it came to rough country. the horse didn't stand a chance.

Back then some of the Tarahumara were still running down game. As more outsiders moved into the area, their territory got smaller and game less plentiful so they turned more and more to subsistence farming, much like our own distant relatives. Now tourists are coming into the area. Copper Canyon is deeper than our Grand Canyon, and people can now get there by train. Genetically, the Tarahumara are the same people as the Pima Indians in Southern Arizona. With the introduction of pickup trucks and supermarkets to the Pima, they now have the biggest problem with obesity and diabetes of any group of people in the nation. This problem didn't exist 80 years ago. You have to wonder how long before "civilization" catches up with the Tarahumara also.

How could they run like that? In addition to the physical characteristics listed above, the lack of fur and those unusual sweat glands also give the human being a big leg up. It's a simple matter of natural air conditioning. When animals covered with fur and/or a thick hide start running, they can start to overheat even in a cool environment. But not you. You start to sweat, which evaporates as you run. And with evaporation comes cooling so you don't overheat. Of course, all of those muscles and tendons that you have developed over time do their job also. So you may end up sweaty and tired, but you also end up with dinner.

Killing For Fun And Profit

Now let's add another important factor: slaughter. Here is my guess: Only a couple of hundred thousand years ago our many hundred times great-grandfather killed something. Remember, flesh and fats were then, and still are today, the gold standard when it comes to energy per mouthful. Let me ask you, if you had to choose to eat just one specific kind of food for the next year what would it be? Wheat, broccoli, corn, or fatty meat? The best choice would be fatty meat. Yes, the vegan crowd may have a fit, but the fact is that if you are told you can only have a single type of food to eat all year, you had better pick fatty meat.

So your very distant relative killed something. So what? Well, maybe he also had a brain just big enough to not only grasp the concept of killing for food — that was fairly standard, but he carried it a step farther. He learned how to hunt that food better than had been done before. But he had a problem: Most other predators had large claws, fangs, and powerful muscles. And so that is when sharp sticks, heavy rocks, and clubs came into play. The sticks probably got longer and sharper and the clubs heaver. When educators write our human history for school children, they say the big thing is that we were "tool makers." What they don't mention is that most of those "tools" were weapons or tools designed to work on the meat or hide produced by those weapons.

And then along came a major invention that would mark a big change in the human position on the food chain. There must have been some Einstein types around back then, and one of these noticed that some broken rocks had sharp edges. And the next big step was learning how to break those rocks so that they had both a point and sharp edges. And from this came the AK-47 of the Stone Age, the stone-tipped spear. This high tech weapon produced more food to feed more people.

This may be oversimplified, but there are at least two places, as mentioned at the first of this, where you can find similar reasoning. In Professor Deirdre Barrett's book

Waistland, the subtitle is *The (R)Evolutionary Science Behind Our Weight and Fitness Crisis*. She also writes about our killer ancestors and their evolutionary dietary preferences. Then she adds today's problem: "Evolution hasn't had time to program us with adaptive signals about how to handle fast-food chains and candy shops." Another place where this running skill is examined is in the study mentioned before by Dennis Bramble from University of Utah and Daniel Lieberman from Harvard entitled *How Running Made Us Human*. They give a very detailed description of the physiology involved.

So generation by generation, our ancestors got smarter and more aggressive because it paid off best. Smarter meant bigger brains. And it is here, the big brain, where they finally hit the wall. But it wasn't "he" it was "she." Bigger brains meant bigger skulls. That skull got big enough that it started to kill women in childbirth. The birthing event for our close primate relatives is a much easier process. Not humans. Our head is so big that getting through the birth canal is a major feat. So the head, and in it, nature's most complex device ever developed, the human brain, had hit its limit. But by then we had become one smart, meat-eating, killing machine.

On The Road Again

Outside of making a defensive argument for the Mafia, what's the point? Just this: As hunters we were not restricted to the tropical zone or its boundaries like other primates.

Those primates had to stick close to that kind of climate because it contained their year-around food supply. As hunters we were free to roam where ever we could find game. And roam we did. And at long last we start to get back to diet.

We call those early people hunter-gatherers. The popular version of this is that these kind, simple folk split up the work. The men hunted while the women gathered in a wonderful and equal separation of work and responsibility. Afterward, they would gather around the camp fire to equally share their bounty, rub each other with pachouli oil, and sing "Kumbaya." If that sounds true to you, then head up to North Dakota in January, which is about what the climate in Northern Europe would have been like for almost six months of the year back then, and head out to do some gathering. I'm afraid that all you will end up with is a basket full of frost bite.

So, it looks simple. It was pretty much meat most of the time for your ancestors. But up crops another problem. Our hunter ancestors may have gotten killing down pat, but they weren't much on conservation. When they killed most of the game in one area, they just picked up and moved to a better territory. But after a great many centuries, they started to run out of that option. And along came farming.

To be fair, there is another way to look at our background. Although the standard take on this is that we are much the same genetic person as our cave man relatives, we might also consider the following: If it was just a matter of random selection, then there wasn't enough time for much change. But what if the selection wasn't all that "random?" For the last several hundred generations, ever since becoming a farming culture, mate selection became a behavior controlled by the elder relatives of the group. This was no minor matter. It took healthy people to work a farm, protect the crops, or fight off those that wanted what you had. To get these healthy children, it took healthy parents. So the selection became of vital interest to all concerned. These healthiest young people would be the ones that could better digest this new carbohydrate and their pairing could substantially speed up the standard evolutionary model.

And grain was something completely new to human diet. Consider our genetic heritage when it came to food. Back before we had learned to be excellent hunters, our bodies were used to primarily a plant-based diet. But this did not include grains. Animals that subsist on grasses and grains have a digestive system far different from our own. Which could account for the fact, as we found out from grave studies, that these first farmers were our sickliest relatives. But they survived. And the ability to digest grains, which they had learned to make more digestible by grinding and cooking, was also part of building a human that could not only survive but even prosper on this new diet.

Another factor that could have accelerated change was the diseases that are associated with the eating of a grain-based diet. In the last few years, research has started to suggest that the gluten in grains may be more of a problem then we had recognized before. Until only recently, it was believed that celiac disease, which is caused by eating gluten and can be deadly to some people, was very rare. But current research has shown that it is more common. Also, the research of professor Alessio Fasano at the University of Maryland's School of Medicine indicates that other autoimmune diseases may also be involved.

But what about those people from that early farming culture who had only a mild reaction to gluten? Here is a guess. In these people, could the eating of gluten confuse the "body brain" and could it have responded by turning it into fat? This would have been a plus if food was scarce and it could be several days to the next meal. If this conjecture is true, it might provide a good reason for those people to survive and be part of our genetic heritage because this fat accumulation could be an advantage if food was limited as it often was. And if this is what happened, wouldn't they be good candidates for those among us today that are now called carbohydrate-sensitive? The same people that have the most trouble with weight gain?

We know this early change to agriculture wasn't the healthiest move our ancestors ever made. But after you kill off most of the game, it beats starvation. However, it brought with it a great many of its own problems. Professor Barrett points out that "The earliest farmers had the worst record for illness and lifespan in human history." In the book *Against the Grain: How Agriculture Has Hijacked Civilization*, author Richard Manning gives a detailed description of the problems. Also Professor Jared Diamond, from UCLA Medical School, wrote an article several years ago regarding the switch from hunter-gathering to farming. The title of the paper was "The Worst Mistake in the History of the Human Race."

The next important step for our ancestors was to start to domesticate, or at least semi-domesticate, wild animals such as cattle, reindeer, sheep, goats, pigs, and about anything else that could provide them with meat and fat, which improved their health and with it their ability to multiply.

So Where Are We Now?

Where do we stand today? There are several answers. For example the diets that are recommenced both by most Departments of Nutrition as well as the United States Government's Dietary Plan come close to those early farmers' diet. There are a number of questions regarding this way of eating, as we have seen in the books that we have examined. There are some people with rather impressive credentials who don't agree that this is even close to the best diet. Where did all of this come from and why is it so strongly defended is where we go next.

Where do we go to get the knowledge we need to develop a healthy diet? Getting the answers needed will turn out to be far more difficult then you might think. Let's start with the Departments of Nutrition themselves. Most of these grew out of the old Home Economics Departments of bygone days. Having visited colleges and universities for over forty years, I can let you in on an open secret: There are some departments that are intellectually rigorous — Chemistry, Physics, Mathematics — and there are others, like the Departments of Education, for example, that are . . . Let's just say that, if you made it through junior high school, you wouldn't find much of a challenge in any of these courses once you have learned the jargon.

I mention the Departments of Education because they often have a direct connection to the Departments of Nutrition. Let me add a bit of history that has to do with how these departments got started. Back in the early 1900s, John Dewey, probably the biggest name in American education, was teaching at Columbia University and in a effort to upgrade American education applied, as was required, to the American Association of University Professors (AAUP), for permission to award a Ph.D. in education. At the time, this was a standard procedure. It involved the AAUP initially sending a general review committee, which was then followed by more specialized groups to perform the multiple evaluations necessary.

154

Years ago I spoke with a professor at the University of Colorado who was a member of that first committee. This person told me that they had barely started their evaluation before it became apparent that this department was lacking the rigor for even a masters degree let alone a PhD. They met with Dewey and expressed their concerns. To the surprise of the committee, he agreed! But he argued that if the level of American education was to be up-graded, the degree was necessary to gain respect. They pointed out that he had the cart several miles before the horse, and the committee left. Dewey, however, was not deterred. He went ahead with his "doctoral program" and rather than a PhD, called the end product a Doctorate of Education.

And so this department is often much maligned, but Dr. Dewey had a point. The Departments of Education that are found in almost all of our colleges and universities are unlike most of the other departments because they are basically trade schools. They are training people to go out and perform a much needed job — teaching.

Why are we looking at this background on the Departments of Education? Because in many cases the Home Economics Department grew out of these departments. Their role, when they started, was to train home economics teachers for secondary schools. Later, they also trained graduates for other institutions that needed nutritionists. From there, these departments grew into today's departments of nutrition. While that is not always the correct history for each department, it will work fairly well as a general statement. Many departments have upgraded themselves to the point they are now much closer to science departments in subject content. An excellent example of how some of these departments have moved on from the old "vacuuming-while-wearing-pearls" approach is the work of people like Dr. Willett. Through mass data studies, his Harvard group is building a body of raw data that can be mined by many in the field for nutritional information.

Although these departments are changing, they still hold some of their old hard-core beliefs. One that has gotten stronger is their "world view" belief that some type of semi-vegetarian diet is best for the for entire planet. From a "politically correct" point of view, they are right. The argument for a primarily vegetarian diet is all there. Less pollution, the ability to feed all of the world's people, much better use of land, no killing of our fellow creatures, and more. But the question that is never fully addressed is this: Is this guaranteed to be the best diet for optimum human health? And that is the question we will keep trying to answer.

How Diets Changed And Why

To start, we should note that the major changes in diet over the last 50 years didn't come from these departments of nutrition, the food industry, or the Federal Government. They came in large degree from medical doctors who were treating patients in the real world and this often got them into a food-fight with the above communities. And that is about where it stands today. Taubes does an excellent job of showing us how we got there. We will now keep trying to find out why.

We have looked at the departments of nutrition, so now let's examine some of the other major players in the food business such as food processing companies, agribusiness, and the United States Government. First, let's look at agribusiness and the United States Government because they are tightly intertwined. The Federal Government spends billions of tax dollars every year to subsidize certain food products. Because the government has invested all of that money in these products, their primary interest, as has been pointed out before, is in selling them. This brings up an important point. The Department of Agriculture, the department that produces the Federal Government's diet guidelines, is not committed to general good health, but to selling the things that they spend billions to subsidize. And, as Willett and others have pointed out, this can be seen in their new diets.

Next we get to the food processors. Again we are talking about billions of dollars being spent to process, advertise, and sell products. You can't make a lot of money selling just plain oranges. But take the juice, add a few traces of vitamins and minerals, and then (and this is the important part) add about 90% plain water and call it a health or energy drink. Push the advertising, get a good spot on the supermarket shelves, and you can make a great deal more money then you ever could just selling plain oranges. Probably one of the ultimate examples of how far this can go is the way that some major companies bottled plain tap water, gave it a fancy name, and made millions.

And since everything from bread to pasta sauce is now, as Pollan pointed out, about chemical engineering as much as it is about food, then there are a lot of ways that the people in the processing business can add a little here or take off a little there to take advantage of the current food fads. Healthy? Questionable. Money making? Oh, yes! If you want an excellent example of this take a look at all of the "low-fat" products. This craze ended up causing more problems than it solved. But one big plus was the way it provided a gold mine for the food processing companies.

A recent ironic example of how far this "processing" can go and its effect on what we think of as a simple food is one of the companies that produces potato-chips-in-a-can. This company was able to successfully convince the tax board in Europe that their product did not contain enough potatoes to be taxed as a potato product.

The Professor's Prescription

Let's return to the campus for another quick look at the departments of nutrition approach to diet. I've already covered their origin, so now let's look at the source of many of their basic beliefs. To do this we are going to have to take another quick detour. Anyone reading this who is also familiar with the general attitudes of higher education is going to scream that I am oversimplifying things, and they would be correct. But it would take another long book to come even close to doing this justice. So the following, although simplistic, will serve our needs.

During the Great Depression of the 1930s, radicals on many college campuses started agitating for change. Whether they took their cue from radicals in Europe or other sources, they had an appealing argument: "More power to the people and equality for all." This fight for equality was no small factor. Remember that clear up to the 1960s, segregation was commonplace in many colleges and universities. Entrance was denied to African-Americans, women, Jews and others. And the academics of that time who called themselves "liberals" stood by and let this happen. So by the 1970s they had been pushed aside, and the radicals, who now called themselves "liberals," became the dominant force, particularly in the social sciences and humanities. They also took the reins in the departments of education (read Diane Ravitch's book *Left Back* for an excellent description of all of this) and with them the departments of nutrition.

As mentioned above, although the leaders of this movement may have changed their name to "liberal," they kept their philosophy, which followed a specific agenda. And, for better or for worse, that is what we see today in much of academia. And it is here where problems started to creep in. Multiculturalism was designed to recognize the different cultures in our society and weigh them all equally. But, over time, it too often became a "blame game," in which Western or European cultures were regarded as the bad guys. Respect for the rights of the individual too often became a toxic "political correctness." And the nutrition departments developed an agenda that made diet a political philosophy with regard to the needs of the world's peoples.

And at long last we get back to specific diets. If your guiding tenet is a political philosophy that demands equality for all and applies that to a world-wide eating plan, you have to recommend almost complete vegetarianism. This is the only way the world's population can be fed. There is just no other choice, because to grow enough meat would require too much of the world's resources. So any suggested diet, and I stress, any suggested diet coming out of most of these departments must be primarily based on plant food. And that is where it stands today. If you think that this political position is a minor matter, then you know very little about academia. These battles are hard-fought. Jobs and promotions depend on how well you can protect this philosophy.

This, at times, can produce some rather bizarre behavior. For example, consider a research experiment that was widely reported by the Associated Press, appeared on a number of the top nutritional web sites, and was published in the *Journal of the American College of Cardiology*. This research experiment was done by The Heart Research Institute in Sydney, Australia and lauded by several dignitaries in the field. The research procedure was this: Fourteen people were fed two different kinds of carrot cake and a milk shake. One kind of cake was made with a polyunsaturated fat and one with a saturated fat. You can guess the results. The polyunsaturated fat and refined carbohydrate mix showed no harm in the subjects' blood profile. But the carrot cake made with saturated fat, from palm oil, and a refined carb showed problems. This same sort of "research," which can be found all too often and labeled as "scientific," is badly flawed but widely accepted. It is flawed because what it proved is that saturated fat mixed with a refined carbohydrate is detrimental. And any good high school science student can tell you that if you want to show that saturated fat is the villain, then you have to remove the other factor and feed the subject only saturated fat to complete the study. That is just basic science.

So why would these people, who should know this, write such a report, and why was it so widely quoted? The answer is that although it may fail as good science, it fits the popular academic paradigm which holds that saturated fat is evil. And it is no surprise that the primary source of saturated fat in today's diet comes from animal sources.

An interesting research project was done recently at Harvard University using the Nurses' Health Study. The researchers took information from women between the ages of 38 and 63 regarding their carbohydrate consumption. From this information, they calculated the glycemic load (remember, a high glycemic load comes from foods like white bread, potatoes, white rice, etc.) and followed these women for ten years. The results showed that women who ate the highest glycemic load had almost twice the risk of heart disease as those who ate the lowest. But, strangely enough, you didn't hear a lot about this.

Another place where an interesting argument can be found is in an issue of the magazine *Scientific American*, which contained an article written by Professor Marion Nestle from New York University. She has also written several good books on diet and its larger ramifications. The article, "Eating Made Simple," pointed out the confusion regarding what to eat. In the first paragraph she states that: "Nevertheless, basic dietary principles are not in dispute: eat less: move more: eat fruits, vegetables and whole grains: and avoid too much junk food." Although this is good general advice, there are those that would take issue with her statement that "basic dietary principles are not in dispute:"

Dr. Nestle has written widely on several aspects of diet and her book *Food Politics*, revised in 2007, is well worth reading, as is her 2006 book, *What to Eat*. Another good read is her latest offering, *Pet Food Politics*, in which she examines the relationship of food supplies for humans, farm animals, and pets and the failure at all levels of food regulation. Some of the points that she makes in the magazine article are of significant interest. For example she points out that food companies prefer studies of a single nutrient because it can then be used to help them sell their products. (You will remember that Pollan made this same point.) She gives the example of adding vitamins to candy and selling it as health food. She is also quite even-handed in some of her observations. For example, she points out the need for calcium in the diet to produce strong bones. But she then notes that this probably depends on more than just the consumption of calcium-rich products because studies have shown that osteoporosis is highest in countries where people consume the most dairy foods. Also, although she is not a fan of eating much meat, she does point out that studies in developing countries demonstrate major health improvements when growing children are fed even small amounts of protein. Dr. Nestle, like some others in her field, is not a great fan of the government's diet plan. She calls it "a disaster."

Included in this issue of the same magazine is an article by the science writer Paul Raeburn regarding a study done at Stanford University (the longest ever done, up to that time) to compare the effects of different types of diets. They compared Atkins, The Zone, Ornish and a standard low-fat diet. The winner was Atkins, with not only more weight loss but also no ill effects on cholesterol.

The Medical Community

Before I get too carried away with any criticism here, I should point out that the reason that many of us are still around today is due to the hard work and excellent research done by these people. But I'm also sure that the good ones in this field would readily admit that there have been past mistakes.

For example the treatment of the lower digestive tract disease diverticulitis. Not too many years ago the recommenced treatment for this condition was a very bland diet. It took several years and further research before it changed to exactly the opposite — a diet rich in roughage.

In the field of cardiology, before the early 1970s, the standard belief was that the best approach for heart problems was bed rest. Then a doctor in Spokane, Washington named

Marcus DeWood took another approach. He inserted catheters into the heart arteries to deal with blockage. This was met with great criticism and some even called it too risky and unethical. But, in only a few years, this approach to blockages became standard. It is a procedure that is done hundreds of thousands of times each year which, with the develop of new drugs and the procedures developed by people like the heart surgeon Michael DeBakey, have saved many lives.

There were doctors up to the 1960s who still held that children, due to undeveloped nervous systems, did not feel much real pain. This belief has always seemed strange to me. When these doctors were children, hadn't they ever fallen off of a bicycle or stubbed a toe? I list this because it is an excellent example of how a belief, even an obviously strange one, can stand for years.

Another popular behavior that can be questioned is the way many doctors still treat fever. Over two thousand years ago the famous Greek physician Hippocrates wrote that fever was a great aid in curing illness. Over the last 50 years, work has been done with both animals and people that shows fever is a major tool that the body uses to fight disease. But there are things that come with fever that we see as problems. We feel poorly. We don't care about eating or doing much. This is what the body is after. It wants you to rest and give it a chance to use fever and its other defenses to fight off the illness. But here is the problem: You, or your sick child, goes to your family doctor with a fever. You want him to do something to make you feel better. He gives you something that lowers the fever. You, or your child, "feels better," and you are sure that the medication helped to "cure" your problem. It didn't. Research has shown it did just the opposite. It probably prolonged the disease. But if you were the doctor, what would you do?

One piece of common advice heard from both doctors and nutritionists is to drink eight 8-ounce glasses of water a day. But there is absolutely no scientific evidence for this recommendation. In an interview with the *Nutrition Action Health Letter*, Dr. Heinz Valtin, Professor Emeritus of Dartmouth Medical School, tells of how he spent almost a year with the help of a professional librarian to evaluate everything available on the subject. Nowhere could they find research that verified this belief. The idea of drinking this much water apparently came from a paper, published back in the 1940s by the Food and Nutrition Board of the Institute of Medicine, which gave this a ballpark estimate as to the amount of liquid needed from all sources. They say that much of this comes from the food we eat. Dr Valtin points out that even white bread can contain 30 percent water. That the companies that sell bottled water have pushed this idea should come as no surprise. Also, he points out that many people believe that coffee, tea, or any drink with caffeine doesn't count because caffeine is a diuretic. The fact is that caffeine is a diuretic only in large amounts and the amount found in popular drinks is too small to have an effect on hydration. Another piece of popular medical advice concerns Vitamin D. Current research has shown that many people don't get enough of this vitamin. To correct this you now hear many of the experts suggesting "15 minutes a day, two or three times a week in the sun, without sun screen." This is a wonderful example how a "one size fits all" approach probably doesn't fit anybody. Compare sun exposure in Florida to that in Maine. Also, we need the help of the body's natural oil to make this work. If you bathe regularly you wash away that oil. So it looks like the best bet is a supplement.

I mention these factors to show how once beliefs are in place they can be very hard to change and for good reason. Mistakes made by most of us are an inconvenience. In the medical profession they can be disastrous. For this reason, coupled with the frequency of legal problems, doctors are forced to stick to prescribed methods of treatment. They have little choice.

Which brings us to the standard medical prescription for weight loss. Most doctors, if asked about weight loss, will prescribe one of the standard calorie-restricted diets. And the result will almost always be the same: The patient will lose weight for the first few weeks. Then, without any cheating on the low-calorie food plan, he or she will stop losing weight and may even gain a pound or two. If the doctor believes the patient (they usually don't), a greater restriction of calories is prescribed. The patient is now constantly hungry but perseveres. A small weight loss follows but finally even this stops. At that point, the vast majority of the time, the patient just gives up. The doctor will attribute the failure to the patient's lack of willpower, not to the fault of the diet plan. And doctors stick to this plan, which in the long run fails over 96% of the time, for the very simple reason that it is cast in stone by the departments of nutrition, where the medical profession must go for their information on diet. So despite its failure, it is the only diet that they feel safe in prescribing.

But as we saw when we examined some of the above books, there are changes that are starting to take place. For example, in a recent issue of the publication *Harvard Health Letter*, Dr. Walter C. Willett made the surprising comment that he thought perhaps that "saturated fat isn't the terrible poison that some have made it out to be." Over the next ten years you may start to see a more moderate attitude to all kinds of fat and more emphasis on good or bad food combinations.

Another example of changing attitudes can be found in a publication from the same institution called *Foods That Heal* (a title that sounds more like a snake oil salesman's pitch than a Harvard publication), in which the authors state: "For many years, it was an article of faith that following a low-fat diet reduced your risk for heart disease and possibly stroke." They then go on to say that the findings from the Seven Countries Study, which was done in the 1960s, showed that people in the region with the lowest incidence of heart disease had the highest percentage of fat in their diet. They also point out that the Harvard Nurses' Health Study, which involved over 80,000 women, showed no relationship between the amount of fat consumed and heart disease.

Please note that the Seven Countries Study that they reference was done in the 1960s. And yet we have been subjected to a constant low-fat mantra for the last 40 years! Why that happened is a question that we will keep examining.

The History of Diet Research

I'm sorry if this gets a bit dull, but we need to examine some background information to gain a better understanding of the confusion surrounding diet. Taubes does a excellent job of covering much of this.

As mentioned before, vehement conflicts over diets are nothing new. In 1865, Banting's diet was admired and attacked, as was Claude Bernard's diet plan in France. In the 1860s, the *Lancet*, then, as now, the major medical publication in England, was quite specific when it said that people like Banting and others "should mind their own business." I mention this because it too often parallels what has happen over the last 50 years in our own country.

Let's start by taking a look at diet advice in the 1950s. As Taubes writes, in 1951, Dr. Raymond Green, along with seven other prominent British clinicians, published a book which advised that people that were obese should adapt an eating plan not dissimilar to that purposed by Banting, Atkins, and others. Even the famous Dr. Spock, whose advice on child rearing sold millions of books, advised that starchy foods were the culprit in weight gain. These were far from isolated proposals. In places like Harvard and Iowa State University in the 50s, Sweden in the early 60s, and the British Obesity Association in an international meeting in Paris in 1971, research showed that carbohydrate restriction in the diet was effective for weight loss.

But then it began to change. In the 1980s, a group of British authorities on diet published *Proposals for Nutritional Guidelines for Health Education*, in which they pointed out that there had been a reversal in thinking and that carbohydrates were not the culprit in weight gain. This change that Taubes calls "one of the more remarkable conceptual shifts in the history of public health" is, by the end of the 1980s, well underway. But even as far back as 1973 the American Medical Association was warning in its publication that the low-carb plan was a "dangerous fad."

Why did this dramatic change occur considering that the basis for this reversal had little in the way of scientific research behind it, and why was it so quickly accepted? Taubes gets right up to this question but never confronts it directly. It's a question that needs to be answered if we are to develop a sensible diet plan.

So Where Do We Go For Answers?

Let's look again at some of the very popular ideas regarding diet:

Let's start with the popular belief that calories in and calories out is the complete answer. Look at what you know from your own personal experience. We all know people who can eat all they want of whatever they want and never gain a pound. And we also know people that seem to be able to gain weight just from breathing. If we want a more documented approach we can look at the many studies done in which volunteers, all of the same age, height, and gender are given a specific number of calories that would be more than needed to maintain their weight. What happens is that they do not all gain the same amount of weight. Which brings up the question, doesn't that raise a bit of doubt regarding the ever popular "calories in calories out" belief?

Perhaps this question has several correct answers. The first would involve metabolism. That metabolism differs from one person to another is obvious. This would mean that food is utilized differently, which would seem to show that different people will have different reactions to the same food.

Also, recent research at the University of Texas Southwestern Medical center involving a hormone called FGF21 could help explain why the low-carb diet could produce weight loss.

The next reason is a bit more complicated. If you reduce the intake of food below what is needed to maintain the present weight of an individual and you keep this up over time, two things will happen. First, the body will use some of its own stores to make up the difference and that person will lose weight. But if the food restriction continues then the body reacts as it has for millions of years. Remember Dr. Lodge's comments on how we talk to the "body brain?" That is what we are doing here. We are telling it that it looks like food will be scarce for awhile and it reacts accordingly. It starts to shut down or restricts the body's use of energy.

If you meet with people that are fasting or have severely restricted their food intake for some time you will notice that while you may be comfortable in shirt sleeves that person will be wearing a sweater. Keeping the body at a pleasant temperature is not a top priority for the "body brain," so it reduces this and other energy expenditures to compensate for the lack of food. Sex will also not be high on that person's "to do" list. There is a group of people that have restricted their food intake for years because they believe it will produce a longer life. This group, called the Calorie Restriction Society, includes people from all over the world who are eating very limited diets. Although the type of food varies, the purpose is always the same: Cut calorie intake to the minimum. They base their behavior on some interesting research that has shown that permanent restriction of calories in a number of animals and insects results in a longer life span.

So you can, if you are highly self-disciplined, keep restricting your food intake to the point that you are only eating a very minimum amount. Over an extended period of time not only will you lose weight but perhaps also extend your life. Again, looking at this from Dr. Lodge's "body brain" point of view, it makes perfect sense. You are telling it that times are bad. It has a very good understanding of this condition because, during the thousands of years of development, this was not an unusual condition, so it knows what to do. It slows down every physical act that it can to conserve the body's energy stores. And why does it wants to keep you around? To replicate itself. As far as it is concerned, this is the whole reason you are here. Over those thousands of years, it has perfected the best ways it can to keep passing on your genes. If you tell it, by limiting food intake, that times are bad, then it will make every effort to keep you around until things get better.

Perhaps another example of how this works is to look at the diet restrictions of the Seventh Day Adventists. This religious group, who are vegetarians, is one of the longest-lived groups in the nation. Again we could ask if this might be the body-brain reaction to the lack of animal protein? In its ancient world, the lack of animal protein meant times were not so good, and it would do what it could to keep you around until things got better. Remember, this is just my guess.

Next we can examine the popular belief that overeating is the cause of overweight, because this would seem to be the case if "calories in and out" is true. In the final analysis the answer would have to be yes, since you can't gain weight from just breathing. But that is a highly qualified yes. Qualified, because the complete answer as to how this works is far more complicated, as we have seen by the writings of several of the authors whose books we have reviewed.

And finally does "calories in and out" work the same for all foods? Research is starting to show the very different reaction the body has to different types of food as well as different food combinations.

A Deeper Look At Why

As we keep seeing, there are many ongoing disagreements, to put it mildly, regarding weight loss as well as the healthiest diet. This question of the healthiest diet can produce some strange results. For example the disapproval of eating meat is not a new aversion. Some of the earlier objections to eating red meat came from the pulpit. It was said that eating it could inflame the baser passions. That is one of the big reasons why so many of the "good health" plans of bygone days were mostly vegetarian.

A wonderful example of how far, and how financially successful, this could be is "The Sanitarium" which was first started in the early 1900s by a devout Seventh Day Adventist named Sister Ellen White, who, like others of her belief, was a confirmed vegetarian. It was interesting that Dr. John Kellogg, who took it over after it had run into financial problems, built the institution around a strong belief in exercise, a vegetarian diet, lots of enemas using both water and yogurt (enemas are again gaining popularity under the name of colonics), and the evils of all sexual activity. To show his dedication to abstinence, Kellogg spent his wedding night writing about the evils of sexual behavior. He considered masturbation an abomination and said it could lead to illness and even death. He writes: "such a victim literally dies by his own hand." It is safe to say that this philosophy soon fell out of favor. The famous corn flakes that carry the Kellogg name were invented almost by accident as they kept trying to find vegetarian diets that were more palatable. But it was an accident that his brother William K. Kellogg saw as an opportunity and the cereal company he formed made a fortune.

We can look again at Taubes' book for the background that he gives on the work done regarding weight loss studies going back over a century, following the techniques and research up to the 1970s. But this leaves us with a puzzling question. Given that most of the research that was done in the 1950s and 1960s involving weight reduction showed that restriction of carbohydrates could produce weight loss, why were these studies simply ignored in the rush to promote a plant-based diet? Trying to answer that question is going to take us back, once again, to the universities, the food processors, and the United States Government.

Where The Ideas Came From

Let's start with academia. As mentioned before, to get on board the popular political attitude of the day, it is mandatory for this group to always look at a "world view." That this is a noble position is obvious, because if the poor of the world are to escape the ravages of starvation it can be done only by some type of vegetarian diet with a stress on corn, wheat, rice, and other grains. These are important because you get the greatest "calories per acre" this way. Also, these products are easy to transport and can be stored for long periods without spoilage, the same reasons that they became the primary products that made a farming civilization possible in the first place. Meat won't work because it takes too great an expenditure of resources to produce meat compared to grain. Also, the storage problems are more complicated.

This view of how to feed the world's people was championed by most of the big names in the field going as far back as the 1950s. People like Ancel Keyes, possibly the biggest name in the diet field at the time, and others would reject any data that refuted their own theories as to proper diet. And as Taubes points out, this was not a big group. At the time, probably fewer than 25 people were primarily in control of most of the diet and nutrition information sources. By the 1970s, those that held this world view were in a position to control most of the big departments of nutrition as well as the federal dollars for research. This meant that this single view dominated clear up to the present day. As we have seen by some of the above book reviews, there were a few renegades in the field, but their impact was limited by a lack of funds and the inability to publish in the major nutritional journals because these were controlled, in the main, by the "world view" group.

Next we get to the role of the United States Government in regard to diet. As has been pointed out before, the branch of government that is responsible for establishing dietary guidelines is the United States Department of Agriculture. Senator Peter Fitzgerald, who at the time was on the Senate Agricultural Committee, commented that this was "like putting the fox in charge of the henhouse." His point being that USDA's primary commitment was selling all of the agricultural products that are subsidized by the government. The USDA is, as shown above, aided in this enterprise by the food processing industry, which spends billions on promotion and millions on political contributions to try to make sure that things don't change.

We now get to a consideration that has not been discussed at length in any of the diet tomes, but may end up being one of the most important factors when it comes to what people will and won't eat. And this is not the scientific, but the emotional, approach to food selection.

The Emotional Side of Food

A book that has gained some popularity is *Skinny Bitch*, by Freedman and Barnouin, followed by their next book, *Skinny Bitch in the Kitch*. These two books are built around a combination of veganism and vulgarity, combined with some rather questionable information and exaggeration. But this type of vegan rant is far from new. In fact, in a less virulent form, it has been a very influential belief for a number of years. It is distinct from the vegetarian beliefs held by people like Ornish, Pritikin, and others who felt that they had scientific reasons for their approach as well as those in the "world view" group. The ideas that we will examine next are those that, based on emotions alone, combined with a dedicated moral stance, feel very strongly that we should not eat our fellow creatures. This group should not be brushed off lightly as they now hold a very influential position in our society.

As Dr. Lodge pointed out, we have taken a giant step out of nature. And this step has taken us into a pretend world where deer are all like Bambi, rabbits are like Thumper, fish are like Nemo, and bears are loveable characters with picnic basket fixations. From nature programs to cartoons, the message is usually to make animals as human and loveable as possible. Also, cats, dogs, and other animals have become dearly loved members of the family. Most people are horrified to find that there are still cultures that eat dogs, monkeys, horses and other animals that many people feel should be protected.

This anthropomorphism is far from new. But today these "true believers" have taken this in a much more aggressive direction. Stop for a moment and consider the vehement vegan's dedicated beliefs that we should not harm our fellow creatures. Now let's take that to a wildly exaggerated, but still possible, conclusion. Wouldn't some questions come to mind? How about krill? They are living creatures and yet are devoured in the millions by whales. But I have yet to see a tee shirt printed with the message "Save the krill. Feed whales whole grains." And then there's tuna. As others before me have pointed out, there are cans of tuna on the grocery shelves proclaiming the contents as "dolphin safe" but nothing about them being tuna safe. Or, if one wishes to go a bit further with this belief, consider termites. As living things shouldn't they be protected? What about a Cockroach Protective Association?

If one wants to push this all the way past absurdity, then we must consider wanton plant cruelty. Think, if you will, of the mother carrot. She spends her whole life struggling to build up enough energy to produce her children. And when the wonderful day is about to arrive for this joyous occasion she is ripped from her happy earthen home and, in some cases, even eaten raw! So we are left with this strange fact: We glorify the carnivorous dolphin and ignore the pitiful pleas of the mother carrot.

Returning to reality, take a look at what has happened to influence the way we view our food. A good place to start would be with the book *Diet For A Small Planet* by Frances Moore Lappé, which was first published in 1971 and sold several million copies. It is one of those books, like Rachael Carson's *Silent Spring*, that happened to be the right book at the right time to express emerging ideas. The Small Planet book came at a time when the "One World" belief was paramount in the departments of nutrition and when religious beliefs regarding diet were just starting to arrive from India and being embraced by the newly emerging counter-culture crowd. All of these meshed beautifully. This philosophy, everywhere from Ornish to Weil, from PETA to vegan, combined with the unnecessary abuse and cruelty of much modern animal production, has a strong influence on many of us. Combine this with the great distance the vast majority of us have from our food sources, and the "food without a face" refrain is appealing.

This objection to eating any animal products by the more dedicated groups can get quite intense. Public demonstrations, throwing paint on fur coats and pointing out in loud declarative terms that the meat eater's stomach is nothing but a disgusting graveyard, are actions that can be part of this group's behavior. It is fair to point out that much of this is not just about animal mistreatment. Far too often the response to the killing of animals, genetically modified foods, and other areas of diet disagreement becomes more of a source of self- aggrandizement for these people than just a true belief. This, at its worst, can involve destruction of property and threat to human life. Few would disagree that better treatment of food animals should be a social priority. Their mistreatment in slaughter houses and feed pens is a major problem that has been addressed in other countries, and there is no reason that it shouldn't change in the United States. But when carried to the point of property destruction and physical attacks, then it has gone too far.

Back To The Food We Eat

To start, let's look at the foods we want to eat. Remember that caveman relative? Well, there were three things that he craved and would eat as much of as he could whenever he had a chance. They were fats, sweets, and salt. Why were those three things so important? Let's start with salt. Isn't it unhealthy? You are always reading where one medical authority or another says so. Well, not exactly. If you ingest too much salt, like drinking lots of sea water, you die. But did you know that if you could take every bit of salt out of everything that you eat and drink that you would also die? You need to keep a saline balance, which means adding some salt to replace that which you lose naturally. But unless our caveman lived by the ocean, salt was hard to come by. So he developed a craving for things that tasted salty and ate them whenever he could. And he passed this craving on to you. Unfortunately, today we can get salt whenever we want it and so we eat around four times what he did — and probably much more than we need.

And fat? Well, you get more energy bang for your buck from fat than any other food. Whenever the caveman could get some, he ate it. And in his day it was hard to find. But he needed it not just for energy, but because it contained things he couldn't do without and his body couldn't produce itself. So he had a craving for fat and, like any good parent, passed that craving on also.

Sweet? It had a big advantage because it helped him decide if something was good to eat. Very few things that are poisonous are sweet. This was a great piece of information to have, and the sweets that he found in nature had the kind of sugar that his body was used to. And since most of these sweet foods were fruits and berries that were available in the fall of the year and the sugars involved could perhaps help him add a bit of body fat, as it did in other animals, to prepare for winter, this was a big plus. Research has shown that humans are prone to be heavier in the fall and winter.

So you crave these things as well, and the food processing companies are glad to help you get them. Go to your neighborhood supermarket and try to find any processed food that doesn't have at least one of these in abundance; a lot of them have two, and some big winners have all three! An interesting insight into these foods can be found in the book that has been mentioned before, *Waistland* by Dr. Barrett. First she describes some of the animal studies, in which researchers found an interesting response to what could be called "exaggerated objects." The Nobel Laureate Niko Tinbergen, a big name in animal research, did some work in this area that might give us some good insights into our own behavior. In his study animals showed a strong preference for artificial objects over the real thing if they were bigger or brighter. For example mother birds would try to feed a fake baby bird mouth rather than their own chick if the mouth was larger than the others. Also some mother birds would ignore their own eggs and try to hatch an artificial egg that was bigger and brighter. Tinbergen called these objects "super-normal stimuli."

So how does that apply to human diet? Dr. Barrett also refers to highly refined food as fitting into the category of super-normally stimulating. It is pretty obvious that the processed food industry discovered this a long time ago. Cake, cookies, pizza, potato chips, and many other foods hold a special place in our food preferences. Dr. Barrett points out that "There is growing evidence that sugary foods can trigger changes in the same brain chemicals that are affected by addictive drugs."

Another place to look for more information regarding the addictive characteristic of some foods is *The End of Overeating: Taking Control of the Insatiable American Appetite*, by Dr. David Kessler. He points out how, for years, the food processing industry has worked diligently to develop products that play on our desire for fat, sweets, and salt. You need only look at a great many of the food products on the market today to see how successful they have been. But because these foods have been developed with the cheapest, and often with synthetic components, this can result in two undesirable results: First, these products contain far fewer of the nutritional components that normally would be found it the natural products that they imitate. And second, chemicals and additives are used to produce the taste, aroma, and mouth feel of a natural food.

But there is a major problem. Our brain and digestive system doesn't get the response of hunger satiation that it would with the real thing. And so it craves more and more trying to achieve this effect. And these cravings are not of minor concern. Almost all of us have cravings that have little to do with real hunger. If you examine those cravings, you will usually find that they involve a product that contains salt or fat or sugar or some combination of these as well some other refined carbohydrates and chemicals to enhance taste.

That products have been developed to produce a craving that borders on an addiction is getting more study from the scientists. Some of the latest functional magnetic resonance imaging (fMRI) studies indicate that some people's cravings produce the same reaction in the brain as a drug addition. Consider how difficult this situation is for them. If you are addicted to cocaine or heroin, this is considered as a very negative social behavior and a major problem. But if the addiction is food, it seems like the whole world is trying to feed your habit! Fast food outlets everywhere. Food ads on television, magazines, and billboards. Also, there is often little understanding from family and friends or even doctors as to just how debilitating this can be. Many of us exhibit cravings that go far beyond simple hunger. Keep this is mind as we, at long last, try to draw some conclusions.

Examining Some Of The Problems

By now you have heard what many of the top names in the field of nutrition believe is the proper diet for the human being. And it is obvious that there is not the general agreement that some suggest. So let me first describe the problems with trying to find the healthiest plan for the individual. The problem with finding that diet and why those problem exist is the real purpose of this book. It centers around the fact that all of the major players in the field have their own agendas and the good health of the individual is not at the top of their list. Just to review again, those major groups are:

1. The United States Government: The billions that they spend on the production of grain puts them in the mandatory position of actively trying to sell those products.

2. The food processing industry: Again, billions of dollars are at stake, and your good health is not on their list of priorities.

3. Academia: Their "One World" philosophy has a strong moral and political underpinning. But it is designed for the many, not for the one.

4. The Emotional Group. The strong moral and emotional tenor of the times, this might be the largest influence of all.

So this is where things in the diet world stand today. The few people that try to go up against any or all of the above groups have a major uphill battle. The best example of how vicious this can become is illustrated by the attacks on the ideas of Dr. Atkins, the anti-poster boy for many of these groups, which continued even after his accidental death from a fall on an icy sidewalk. A group called "Physicians Committee for Responsible Medicine," which Time Magazine points out is comprised of only 5% doctors (and what kind of "doctor" — medical doctor, naturopath, chiropractor, etc. – is not addressed), even tried to get his medical files released to the public.

To appease the Emotional Group as well as the Academics, diet authors who wanted to take the low-carb approach did so by eliminating saturated fat. The hidden side effect that they look to achieve with this approach is that it takes animals out of the picture. The refrain, "saturated fat is a great evil" contains the hidden message "don't kill animals," which satisfies the agenda of several of the above groups.

A recent book by P. Michael Conn and James V. Parker called *The Animal Research War* does a good job of showing how this has now gone from discussion to violence. They point out that 20 years ago endocrinologists like Dr. Conn would meet with animal rights activists to try to address their concerns. Now a radical wing of this group has become so violent that it is scaring researchers out of the field. This radical group has become so virulent that the FBI now calls them a serious domestic terrorism threat.

To show the strength of these beliefs, consider the following: One of the best-designed and longest-running supervised diet research studies ever accomplished was completed in 2008. The results were published in one of our nation's most respected medical journals, *The New England Journal of Medicine*. Kelly Brownell, director of Yale University's Rudd Center for Food Policy and Obesity, lauded this group of researchers for the quality of this project. One of the big advantages of this study was that the subjects ate in their company cafeteria so a verifiable intake was possible, which is a big problem with many studies. It is usually a problem because, as I have said before, the three things people lie about most are money, sex and food. Also the number of researchers per subject was far greater than normally found. There were 23 researchers involved in supervision and observation of the two-year study, which included 322 moderately obese subjects divided into three groups. The first group was put on a low-fat, restricted calorie diet (1500 calories for women and 1800 for men). The second group was put on a Mediterranean diet with the same calorie restrictions. The third group was put a low-carbohydrate, Atkins type diet with no calorie restrictions.

Notice the calorie limit for the first two diets, which is about the standard calorie count for the average slow weight-loss diet. Also, again, note that the low-carb diet had no calorie restriction. The results? Those on the low-carb, no restriction diet lost slightly more weight even without restrictions. But the biggest surprise was that their cholesterol results were the best of all three groups!

Because we have been told for years that one of the big problems with a low-carb diet was the negative effect it would have on cholesterol, shouldn't this have been big, exciting news? Also shouldn't it be newsworthy that they had no restrictions on how much they could eat and still lost weight? It wasn't. In fact it garnered some rather strange comments. For example, Gary Foster, director of Temple University's Center for Obesity Research, was quoted in an article by Sally Squires, from the Washington Post, as saying, "From a weight-loss perspective, it all comes down to calories."

In a report from *ABC News* on their website, Dr. Meir Stampfer, co-chair of Brigham and Women's Hospital in Boston, said "it proves the low fat diet is not necessarily the best diet." He added, "The low-carb and Mediterranean diets are good as long as the protein and fat sources are healthful." These are, of course, the standard code words for "no animal fat." ABC's medical editor Dr. Timothy Johnson has said he was "amazed at all the hoopla" regarding this study. He goes on to add that the weight loss was "no big thing." Dr. David Katz, director of the Prevention Research Center at Yale, says that the study "highlights that weight loss can be achieved in a number of different ways," and then adds, "and be sure to control calories." Why, in the face of this type of information, would they continue to make comments that don't fit the data? I think part of the reason is that they have seen the vehemence of the "true believers" when their beliefs are challenged. We could keep going over study after study but the results keeps coming out the same.

Some of the latest studies are even more telling. A huge study out of Harvard University this year looked at the eating habits of 1.3 million people in regard to eating beef and pork. They could find no relationship with eating these foods and heart disease. Another study out of Stanford University called the A to Z Study (Atkins to Zone) showed again that the Atkins approach produced the greatest weight loss and also the best improvement in cholesterol. However, the latest study out of Harvard says that there is a health problem with red meat.

So, at last, let's ask the obvious question: Why do we keep getting these responses when the data shows otherwise?

The problem, I think, comes down to this: The Federal Government, the food processing companies, the majority of academics, as well as those with an emotional agenda, are all locked into one over-reaching approach. Those with a differing opinion are either attacked or ignored. To my knowledge, there is no "Carnivores Protective Association" that champions a meat-eating point of view. We have looked at some of the books by those individuals that do, and there is no doubt that they are starting to have more influence, but an honest and open debate on the subject of diet still seems to be in the future. There is a old saying that knowledge advances on funerals. There is a lot of truth in that statement. If you have spent your life developing one specific position and your reputation is based upon it, then you will fight long and hard against change.

One last comment on the emotional approach to diet. This is now stronger than any other belief regarding food, because, when everything is considered, it just sounds so much kinder. It is true that you won't find people at the better eating places bending over their steak and asking for forgiveness before picking up a knife. But as the world we live in becomes more and more artificial our society responds best to the invented "feel good" concepts followed very quickly with "We are right, and you are not just wrong but a bad person." We can do this because we are almost completely insulated from the natural world when it comes to food. I do not submit that this is all bad. You need only read a book like *Slaughterhouse* by Gail Eisnitz to agree that there should be changes. But when popular beliefs — don't eat fat, we must not kill other animals, radical veganism — start to promote violence as well as provide a potentially negative impact on human health, it would seem that people in positions of authority in the field would take a much more objective view. Far too often that has not happened.

If you could walk into an average third grade classroom and ask, "How many of you think we should kill and eat other animals?" I can assure you that few if any hands would be raised. If, however, you ask the same group, "How many of you like to eat hamburgers?," most hands would shoot into the air. This happens because this strange separation from nature has now become the norm. As we move farther and farther away from nature, this emotional approach continues to become more popular simply because it makes us feel that by this behavior we are the "good guys." If this trend continues to gain strength you have to wonder if it will go the way of prohibition in the 1930s. Will you have to knock on a door in a dark alley and give the password to get into a steak house restaurant?

At Long Last, The Reason Why

Over the last 40 years we became the fattest nation in the industrialized world because the major authorities have made the word "FAT" the most frightening word in our nutritional vocabulary. Non-fat and low-fat products became king on our market shelves. Our general population was sold again and again on the belief that eating fat was a bad thing. When it all started forty years ago, this was the message that was stressed over and over by government, academia, and food companies. And this advice became the norm and was accepted by most of our population. Next came "some fats are good," but this never got the heavy publicity of the "Bad Fat" mantra.

And that is the main reason that we are a fat nation! There is a graph in Dr. Willett's book that shows how. Over time, as our fat intake decreased, our body weight increased. Why? Because fat in the diet gives hunger satisfaction. Without it we simply have to eat more to feel full. Yes, there are other factors that have changed during that time period, but the big reason is that "fear of fat" remains the big factor in the nation's diet.

So At Long Last Some Diet Suggestions

After reading all of the above it only seems fair that at this point this book should reveal a "Super diet." It, of course, would have to have a catchy name as well as promise that it would solve all of your weight problems in only a matter of weeks, with little effort on your part. I'm sorry, but my suggestions won't even come close. I should also stress that I have neither the professional training nor medical degrees necessary to prescribe even a breath mint. All I have done is use the research of others to try to reach some possible conclusions. And let me stress again, I am only presenting possibilities, not prescriptions.

Almost all diets work. But the vast majority of the time,

they represent only a temporary fix. Why does it happen that way? To show why, let's consider how other approaches to other problems work. A good example is our approach to curing illness. When you are sick with the flu, a cold, or most of the other common illnesses, it runs a predictable cycle. The illness gets worse until you reach what is often called the "crisis," at which time the body develops the means to fight it off and you start to recover. Let's say that just before the crisis, when you are feeling your worst, you go to see a medical doctor, a faith healer, a voodoo priest, a naturopath — or you start using grandma's famous cure. You pass the crisis and start to recover. You are now a true believer in any of the above "cures" because you are convinced that it was what worked. A new book, *Tricks or Treatment* by Simon Singh and Edzard Ernst, does a wonderful job of showing that almost all of the alternative medicines that make up a $77 billion industry are bogus. They wonder "why so many people spend so much money on such transparent quackery."

In a way, this happens with any diet. When you start out, you now watch what you eat. You are careful to stay on the plan, and you start to lose weight. But then something happens: A party at work, a special night out, dinner at a friend's house — and you cheat on your diet. This breaks the diet pattern, and you stop being so diligent about what you eat. So you start to gain the weight back. And here is the interesting part: you don't blame the diet, you blame yourself!

Was it your fault? Yes and no. Obviously yes, because you failed to follow the diet. But because this was a generic "one size fits all" type of plan, which is the mainstay of almost all of the popular diets, it didn't specifically fit you. And this second statement isn't original but is probably the most important: No "diet" is ever going to solve your weight problem. You already know the answer to all of this. It is simply that you are going to have to permanently change what and how you eat.

No, it is a long way from a new idea, but it is a decision that you have to make before any eating plan will work. It is sad but true that information about diet is too often the product of politics, profit, or emotion and not hard science. And so you will have to think carefully as you build your own plan because it will be with you for life.

Let's start by again looking at some of the most popular types of diet. The big three are some type of low-carb diet, a vegetarian diet, and one primarily vegetarian but including some of fish and chicken with a stress on fats other than the saturated ones, which is often called the Mediterranean Diet. We have looked at these from several angles and by now you have some idea of what might fit you best. Don't rush into this. If you are part of a couple or have a family whose needs will have to be considered, this will take some discussion. This looks like it could be a problem but it could end up being a help. Tell your partner and/or your family what you are planning to do and ask for their help working out the details. It would be best, if you can, to design a plan of healthy eating that gets everyone on board.

As you build your own diet plan consider the following food groups:

Proteins. This is a big decision because of the different types and choices. If you go vegetarian this will take a bit of research and planning. Any good vegetarian cookbook will show the food combinations that are needed to provide this nutrient. Let me admit to a bias here. Given our genetic history, I am a strong believer in the protein in red meat, pork, fish, chicken, etc. as an important part of human diet. Vegetarians will cry foul and vegans will scream invectives, and they have a point. But we still have a lot to learn about all kinds of protein. And right now, as Willett pointed out, we know the minimum amount of protein that is necessary but we can't say with scientific conviction that how much is needed for good health, or even of what type.

The big problem with eating any animal protein is the way that this type of product is raised and handled. The major producers of beef, pork, and chicken not only can be criticized for the cruel way these animals are often treated but for the problems, from a health point of view, that arise from the hormones, antibiotics, and other additives that are fed to some of these animals. One answer to this problem is the growing number of places where organic alternatives are available. There is another problem that influences the selection of a protein-based diet. Do you remember that Dr. Sears in his book *The Zone* said that the problem with this diet is that it changes the composition of the fat on our bodies? I have not seen others in the field agree with this, but it may be a problem. From what I have heard from people on this plan when they first tried the Atkins diet it was a great success. However, when they went back to their old way of eating, they gained the weight back. And here is the problem: Every time they did this it became harder and harder to lose the weight. From the body's point of view, it would make sense. It will do everything in its power to hold onto fat. For all of its evolutionary past, fat meant survival. By going back and forth, you are making it learn how to hold onto fat a new way. Remember this is all a guess on my part as I have not seen any test data to show that this is what happens.

Carbohydrates. For years we heard about good and bad fats. Now we are hearing more about the good and bad carbohydrates. There are some people who have trouble with certain members of this group due to allergies or genetic problems such as celiac disease. But let's start with the above-ground vegetables. Most people can eat their fill of red, green, and yellow vegetables and not have any problem with weight gain or allergies. If your plan is to lose weight, then there are things in this group that should be carefully examined. Refined grains and sugars are serious problems for many people and probably should be avoided as much as possible if you are trying to lose weight. As mentioned before, a study done recently at Harvard, using data from the Nurses' Health Study, pointed to problems with a high-carbohydrate diet. Using the glycemic load as an indicator they found that those in the highest glycemic load group had a higher risk of developing heart disease than those in the lowest group. Remembering that the highest glycemic load comes from things like refined grains, potatoes, white rice, and many sweeteners, it would seem prudent to limit the inclusion of these foods. Remember this: It is hard to gain weight without eating carbohydrates. So select these carefully.

One of the problems with eating vegetables is similar to the one with eating meat. The use of different types of chemicals and poisons to force faster and larger growth as well as to protect against insects can be a real concern for the consumer. The Center for Disease Control has expressed concern regarding the levels of several chemicals beginning to be found in our population. Here again an organic approach seems to address many of these problems.

Fats. Here is where we get into very uncertain ground when it comes to diet. We have looked at the books by those that think fat is evil and those that don't. Current research does show that our bodies need some fat for good health. The question is how much and what kind? There is no safe scientific answer to this as yet, so this is a question you will have to decide for yourself. However, Dr. Willett recently has suggested that the amount in a good diet could be as high as 40 percent. The big advantage of including different kinds of fat in your diet is that when combined with protein it does an excellent job of controlling hunger. The problem with saturated fat shows up most when it is combined with a refined carbohydrate.

Fruits and nuts. This is listed as a separate nutritional group although it is a combination of some of the above. A number of the books we have looked at warn how fruit can kill a diet. If you have had problems with losing weight it would probably be wise to hold off on fruit, as well as nuts. But as soon as you can, I would start adding back a few nuts followed by fruit when you hit your desired weight, because of the nutrients they provide.

Eggs, Milk and Alcohol. This sounds like the start of an eggnog recipe, but it's nothing that exciting. Without exception, all diet recommendations exclude all kinds of alcoholic beverages during the weight-loss phase and for good reason. Alcohol's ability to produce weight gain far exceeds its calorie content. Perhaps it is because it is absorbed into the system directly through the stomach wall, which makes it look like a "super carb" to the body.

Milk has its own problems for many people. Most of us lose the ability to digest milk by the time we reach puberty, and for some this can cause real digestive problems. The recommendation seen in the Federal Food Pyramid for dairy consumption are questioned by several of the people in the field. Willett points out that there are better sources of calcium. The primary argument for consumption is that it helps build strong bones. This may well be true, but studies have shown that some of the societies with the highest dairy consumption have the highest rate of osteoporosis. The "why" of that isn't clear but it brings the often-heard argument for dairy consumption into question.

For a time eggs were regarded as undesirable due to their cholesterol content. Most authorities have backed away from this restriction. The amount of cholesterol eaten by most people has little effect on cholesterol in the blood as the body can adjust to its needs by increasing or decreasing the production from the liver. For these people, eggs do not present a problem. For the few for whom eating food containing cholesterol does increase the amount in the blood, the amount of eggs should probably be limited. However, eggs are one of nature's excellent foods, and if they are not a problem for you, can be highly recommended.

Exercise. No, this also isn't a food group but it is just as important as anything you eat. There simply is no choice here. You will have to plan on reaching a goal of at least 30 minutes a day as a minimum, five or six days a week. If you are trying to lose weight, then an hour a day would be even better. But if you are not used to exercising, it is important to start slowly. Exercise is a deal-breaker for many people. But consider this: If you want to eliminate up to 70% of the diseases and disabilities that are waiting for you down the line, then there is simply no other choice. As we have seen in several of the books reviewed above, up until only a few years ago, many of the diet professionals didn't suggest much of anything in the way of exercise. An example of the change in attitude can be seen in the Ornish books. In his first book, he is not much of a fan. But in his second book, he says it is necessary.

You see this change in almost all of the newest diet books as well as in the research that is finally being done in the field. For example, look at a study started in the 1980s at Stanford University that involved 538 middle-aged runners. One of the purposes of this project was to show how, over time, this kind of physical activity would produce problems with feet, knees, and back as well as a have a negative impact on longevity. (This belief illustrated the attitude of many in the field at that time.) The results were just the opposite. Many of those involved in this project were "surprised" at this outcome. And this is only one example, from many, that could be cited, that show the positive results of exercise. If you have any doubt as to its benefit read the opinions of either Willett or Lodge as to its necessity.

The key to a good exercise plan is to start at a level that you can easily achieve. This means taking into account your age and physical condition. If you are over 60 and haven't exercised since high school, don't make the big mistake of thinking that pushing yourself hard is a good plan. Pushing too hard too soon is the source of many of the problems that are associated with exercise. Starting with something fairly easy and building on it is the key to a good program.

Remember you need two types of exercise: cardiovascular and resistance training. Look over the number of books that are out there on exercise and plan carefully. Some of the best plans include resistance training two or three days a week in addition to cardiovascular workouts. But remember, the secret to success here is do not push yourself too hard to start. Start out slowly and just keep increasing until you reach the goals that you have set for yourself.

The most common objection to an exercise plan is simply finding the time. After family and job, there often seem to be just too few hours in the day. Look at it this way: Let's say that your doctor calls you and says that your last physical showed that you have a type of cancer that calls for immediate surgery and extensive chemotherapy. Would you answer that you just don't have the time right now what with new responsibilities at work and that big vacation the family is planning? No, I don't think that is the way you would handle the problem. But exercise and diet are like that. If you wait until you have the health problems to try and start, then the damage has already been done.

As you plan, remember that you were designed by your biology to be lazy. Your body is not going to be wild about doing anything that uses energy unless it produces more energy or offspring. That you would voluntarily exercise is not in its genetic plan. Because of the body's desire to do nothing as much as it can whenever it can, it means that it will take real dedication on your part to make an exercise program work.

The major problem that most people face when it comes to exercise is the matter of place and time. For some the answer is a gym membership. The advantages of going to a gym is that instructors are usually available to help you get started. Also, you can do this in groups where you help each other to stick with it and achieve your goals. The disadvantages are the cost and the fact that it takes more time. Another approach is to set up your own equipment and develop your own workout program. To start, this takes little more than some light weights and good athletic shoes. If you go this route and live in a climate where snow and rain are a problem, then I would strongly recommend the addition of something like a stair-stepper, a rowing machine, or a ski machine. Sadly, there are a number of these around that have become little more than clothes racks and can be purchased for less than half of the new price.

Your choice of gym or home workout is not a small decision because of the time and money investment involved. And when it comes to time, this becomes a major commitment. There are those that make this a pleasant part of their day because it means meeting with friends and enjoying both exercise and camaraderie. But because you will be doing this five or six days a week it will take a big chunk of time. And if you have a family, a job and other obligations this often can be difficult to maintain.

Working out at home takes less time, but does take some planning and real self-discipline. The best answer for many people is to just accept the fact that you are going to get up and get it done first thing in the morning. Again, this isn't easy. It means getting to bed earlier, getting the TV out of the bedroom, and, most of all, not hitting the snooze button on the alarm clock. If you can just force yourself to do this for 30 days it will often become enough of a habit that you can maintain this plan of action. I am not trying to pretend that you will leap up in the morning, eager to exercise. But I do think that if you get up, get your program completed, and know that you have done much of the exercise needed, it will give you a good feeling to start your day. A minimum of 30 minutes in the morning, a real effort to walk more, to take the stairs when possible and a number of other changes can meet the exercise requirements of most people. But if you are overweight you should work up to around an hour a day.

Finally, keep this in mind: no diet will work if you are hungry all the time. You have to develop a diet that at the end of a meal leaves you satisfied. Here again you have to consider the vast difference between hunger and craving. You have to satisfy true hunger for a diet to work over the long haul. When it comes to craving, that is when you simply have to gut it out. By simple force of will, you have to win this fight. It can be done. "Take it one day at a time" may have become a very old idea, but it is still around because it can work. One positive note: The longer you fight, the weaker your cravings become. It's true. For the first few days it is a major battle. But after the first two weeks you will notice that the craving is not as powerful as it used to be. But be on guard because even months later that craving, without much warning, can come roaring back. But you can win because you must never lose sight of the fact that this is a fight for your life. And that is really is no exaggeration.

Because diets are so common in our culture we too often look at them as simple procedures. They are not. Television, magazine and newspaper advertising as well as most books on the subject often stress how fast and easy this or that diet can be. The books and advertisements that tout this or that program stress the ease of success to sell a product. Very few discuss the real difficulty of changing eating and exercise habits permanently. Consider this: we tend to think that drunks can be funny. Yet alcohol causes more deaths, car accidents, and social problems than any other drug in our society. Tobacco use kills many thousands but we often make fun of the problems involved with quitting. And eating is considered a casual behavior with not much thought involved regarding its level of difficulty.

If you are seriously overweight, look carefully at this problem because it is almost a guarantee that your approach to certain foods has become an addiction. Is this an overstatement? Considering all of the problems that these foods cause you right now and those problems that could be waiting in the future, it may not be that much of an overstatement at all.

And so we get to several very big problems that you will have to consider. If you had an addiction to heroin or cocaine, your friends and family would do everything they could to help you with your recovery. But tell them that you have a food addiction, and most will just laugh or tell you that you are just being overly dramatic. But the fact is that you do have a problem with food if you are seriously overweight. This problem has grown over the years. With each failed diet it gets worse. And this problem keeps getting worse because our society has gotten to the point where one of our great pejoratives is the word "fat." The virulence of people's response to this condition is startling. We long ago made racial, ethnic, and gender slurs unacceptable. But the fat jokes, slurs, and ostracism seem to be regarded as generally acceptable. And so many people get to the point that they are truly neurotic when it comes to the way they regard food.

And so we get to an unpleasant part of dieting that is seldom addressed. For much of the following we will once again use some of the excellent information to be found in Dr. Barrett's book *Waistland*. Remember the discussion involving super stimuli? Step back for a moment and look at the way our society regards the simple act of eating. There are food columns in most newspapers as well as magazines, television shows, and books by the thousands covering the subject. And look at the mystique surrounding "fine dining." It is amazingly easy to spend hundreds of dollars for a four-person dinner at a "fine" restaurant.

Why this tremendous involvement with food? Is this even remotely connected to eating to stay alive? Of course not.

A long time ago the vast majority of people in our nation stopped worrying about getting enough food to live. And the next step was the same one that we took with clothing, cars, homes, and a number of other things that are based on what, a very long time ago, were necessities. That step, from food to fetish, was to make these things a status symbol. This is far from being new. As far back as ancient Egypt or Rome, the rulers indulged in unusual and rare foods, in great part just to show the superiority of their social position. And in many ways this has been passed down to us. To get a good table at an expensive restaurant, to afford a fine wine, to know the latest food fads — and to feel that these things are vitally important — are all too common today in our society.

As Dr. Barrett points out, this is the basis for many eating problems. Almost all diet books will use the majority of their pages giving you recipes for delicious food. In Ormish's latest book he even includes beautiful pictures of food dishes in full color. Most of us don't have any problem at all finding foods that we think are delicious. And that is the basis of much of our problem with overweight. Think about this carefully as you develop your plan. Look at your own "super foods" as a drug to which you are addicted. If you think that this sounds like a gross exaggeration, consider this: If you continue to indulge in these foods that make you fat, they will very likely make you chronically ill or kill you. Obesity is a major contributing factor in diabetes, heart disease, cancer, arthritis, and other health and personal problems.

A drastic approach for some obese diabetics, when all else fails, is surgery. One example is bariatric surgery. In a recent research project, this operation was used on obese diabetics. They lost a substantial amount of weight, which cured the disease in the majority of those involved. But most of us would not care to have a surgeon take a scalpel to our stomach to try to cure a problem that stems from poor diet. There is also a more drastic approach which is more surgically invasive. For some this is their last resort. But keep in mind that these are new procedures. Problems that may happen in the future are simply not known.

And many of these problems of overweight may just be starting. Look at the statistics for the last twenty years in regard to weight gain. The standard chart showing weight gain in our nation, starting with 1981, looks like an ascending staircase year by year. In 1981, the number of overweight people was 8.6%, and the number of those that were obese was 4.1%. By 2000 the numbers were 24.8% overweight and 25.6% obese! Why? There are probably several answers, but two stand out. One big factor was that general activity level dropped. More TV and video games, less outdoor involvement. And, of course, the other was diet. Also an interesting statistic given by Dr. Willett that I mentioned before,and that I have seen elsewhere is a very strong inverse relationship regarding the inclusion of fat in our diet and weight gain. As we started eating less fat we started gaining more weight. And this "eating less fat" which is a product of the "no fat" or "low fat" craze is never examined as it should be. Just look at the statistics. The huge weight gain of our population, over a comparatively short time, has to point to a very major change in behavior of the majority of our population. And it has to be the "anti-fat fad" because nothing else fits the statistics as well. There are other factors but they are minor in comparison. Almost every day we see the small concessions that are slowly moving us away from this destructive fad. But it will happen slowly. There are too many reputations and too much money tied up in the "fat is bad" paradigm to expect those involved to admit that the whole thing was a major disaster.

One major problem that is just coming to light is the increase in strokes and heart attacks in middle-aged women. This would seem to have a direct correlation to the reduction of activity and increase in weight gain. It is interesting that Japan has passed a law that will require that attention be paid to overweight. This from a nation that has one of the world's slimmest populations. Their action has little to do with appearance but everything to do with good health.

But let's get back to your eating plan. Ask yourself if you really are addicted to some foods. The truthful answer is almost always "yes." Stop for just a minute and think about the food or foods that always are the ones that make you go off of your diet. Pizza? Ice cream? Beer? Donuts? And the list goes on. You may have heard people say jokingly, "Oh, I'm just addicted to ice cream." Sadly, it's probably no joke. Ask yourself if you are sure you know the difference between hunger and craving. If you finish a full meal and still want dessert, you have just had a good look at a craving. It is imperative that you identify all of these because once you start to really examine your eating habits there will probably be many more of them than you might think. Much more than you probably realize, you have based far too many of your eating decisions on cravings, not hunger. Look carefully at those foods that could be call your "super foods." I don't think that you will find broccoli or Brussels sprouts on that list. But you will find foods that contain some combinations of things like refined flour, high-fructose corn syrup, sugar, fat, or salt. Not many people in the diet field list flour as a major problem. In fact, whole-grain flour is recommended by vegetarians. But it can cause problems for some people. The book written by Cleave and Campbell, as far back as 1966, showed a problem with combining saturated fat with flour. Their research involved white flour, but I think that even whole grain products produce the same results to a lesser degree. Perhaps we can look again at Dr. Cordain's comment in his book *The Paleo Diet* where he says that when it come to healthy foods, "grains and legumes are marginal at best." Do you remember how the authors of *The Paleolithic Prescription* wrote about finding plaque in the arteries of men in their teens and early twenties? Something in the diet is causing this condition and saturated fat, and of late trans fat, have been called the culprits. But as you can tell from the above, it could be the act of combining these fats with refined carbs that may really be the prime suspect.

Again turning to Dr. Barrett, we find an interesting comparison to raw versus refined. She points out that chewing coca leaves doesn't seem to affect the health of South American natives and poppy seeds aren't usually a health risk. But refine them to cocaine or heroin and the story is much different. She points out that salt, fat, sugar and starch aren't harmful in their natural contexts. But refine these products, and you have the major "problem food" products of today. Do you remember the book, *Neander-thin* that was reviewed? That book, written years ago, proposed an eating plan based on raw foods as much as possible. This idea is coming back into vogue. Although it may take a lot of planning, its big advantage is that it cuts out all processed foods.

Whichever diet you choose don't expect it to be easy. Most diet plans tell you how fast and easy their plan is. If they are, then that is why they are seldom ever a permanent solution. The fact is this: It will be difficult. You will not eat what most people eat. It will be more expensive and time consuming than before. And it will take time to produce the desired results. If you are seriously overweight it could take two years to reach and hold the body weight you want. But I can guarantee you this: Within 60 days you will start to notice a difference. And at the end of two years you will have more energy, feel and look better than you have in years or perhaps ever. You will remember all the hard work and sacrifice that it took to accomplish this, and you will have no desire to go back to the way you were.

Some Last Thoughts

Just how really important is all of this? Research has reached the point where we can now say with a great deal of confidence that most of the chronic conditions that start in middle age could be postponed or eliminated by proper diet and exercise. It is rather sad that the primary reason that most people go on diets is not to protect their health but just so they can look good for swimsuit season. Yes, it is understandable that we all would like to have an attractive appearance, but shouldn't life-long good health really be the major goal?

It is important to understand that small changes just don't work. And it's true that good diet and exercise habits do have their downside. If it were easy, you wouldn't see all of those people waddling down the street. You will eat differently than most people. For example, if you see a product advertised on television, it's a good bet that you shouldn't eat it. Remember Dr. Lodge's simple diet advice: Don't eat crap! Also, as Pollan pointed out, we should go back to eating food and not nutrients. Almost every month some new research shows how this or that nutrient found in this or that product has some wonderful effect. A good example of this would be resveratrol, a component of red wine. When positive results reported in animal studies regarding resveratrol was reported, it caused some in the health field to sing the praises of red wine. What was overlooked was the statement made by the researcher himself that it would require the drinking of 160 bottles to achieve the same amount used in his study. But I think that Pollan was right when he said that what we really should focus on is just getting back to eating good, healthy food. He said that if your grandmother couldn't have recognized it as food you probably shouldn't eat it.

You have heard all of your life about the desirability of a well-balanced diet. I have never heard anyone question this advice. But then look at what is usually touted as well-balanced. The new government diet plan would fit this description, and we have seen again and again how many top names in the diet field don't think that it is even close. The best advice is build your own.

You are starting to hear more and more about the new drugs that are being developed to produce weight loss. Toward the end of one of Oz's diet book he lists a large number of drugs that are in the developmental stage. The reason for all of this activity is obvious. A pill like this could make that drug company billions. But do we really know the long-term effects of fooling Mother Nature? What we do know, without question, is that a healthy diet, rigorous exercise, proper rest, and emotional commitment is a time-tested prescription for a good life and excellent health.

There are four physical conditions in which you can find yourself. They are:

1. Proper body weight and good physical condition.

2. Overweight and good physical condition.

3. Proper body weight and poor physical condition.

4. Overweight and poor physical condition.

Of course, the first condition is by far the best. But failing that, work hard to achieve the second one. But remember if you fit into category three you may look grand in those skinny jeans, but there are probably problems down the road. And if number four describes you, then you have a major problem, and you should do everything in your power to correct it.

Good Luck.

www.ingramcontent.com/pod-product-compliance
Lightning Source LLC
Chambersburg PA
CBHW060247290526
45789CB00001B/235

* 9 7 8 1 4 6 9 9 5 4 7 5 2 *